SMALL WINS
BIG
HEALTH

SMALL WINS
BIG
HEALTH

10 SIMPLE HACKS
to Boost Fitness, Tame Stress, and
Build a Healthier Version of You!

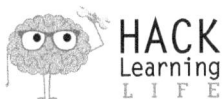

HACK
Learning
LIFE

BRYAN
HOLYFIELD

Cover and Interior Design by Steven Plummer
Project Management by Regina Bell
Editing by Tarah Threadgill
Copyediting by Jennifer Jas

Paperback ISBN: 978-1-956512-59-5
eBook ISBN: 978-1-956512-61-8
Hardcover ISBN: 978-1-956512-60-1

Library of Congress Cataloging-in-Publication Data is available for this title.

First Printing: September 2024

To Hannah.

I do not deserve the love, grace, and joy
you've given me for fifteen years!

CONTENTS

FROM THE PUBLISHER

Introducing the Hack Learning Life Series by the creator of the Hack Learning Series

AFTER ALMOST A decade of helping educators turn problems into solutions, Times 10 Publications applies the same simple-to-follow protocol to the Hack Learning Life Series to help all of us overcome life challenges. Hack Learning Life books center on what you already know and provide shortcuts to make life a little easier—who doesn't need this?

Based on the same practical six-part framework from the Hack Learning Series for educators, Hack Learning Life helps you unpack the problem, identify quick wins, make a long-term plan for success, and overcome the obstacles that may slow you down—all while providing stories from the authors or from people like you, doing the work and finding success.

REBRANDING THE HACKER

A hacker is someone who explores programmable systems and molds them into a different form, often a better one. Hackers are known as computer geeks—people who like to take applications and algorithms to places their designers never intended. Today, hackers are much more. They are people who explore many ideas both in and out of the technology world. They are tinkerers and fixers. They see solutions to problems that other people do not see.

Steve Jobs and Mark Zuckerberg might be considered technology's greatest hackers. No one taught them how to build an operating system or a social network, but they saw possibilities others couldn't see. Hack Learning Life is a collection of books written by people who, like Jobs and Zuckerberg, see things through a different lens.

They are practitioners, researchers, coaches, nutritionists, professionals, and specialists. They live to solve problems whose solutions, in many cases, already exist but may need to be hacked. In other words, the problem needs to be turned upside down or viewed from another perspective. Its fix may appear unreasonable to those plagued by the issue. To the hacker, though, the solution is evident, and with a little hacking, it will be as clear and beautiful as a gracefully designed smartphone or a powerful social network.

INSIDE THE BOOKS

Hack Learning Life books are written by passionate people who are trained experts in their fields or longtime practitioners offering experiences that most readers do not have. Unlike your typical how-to books, Hack Learning Life books are light on research and statistics and heavy on practical advice from people who have experienced the problems about which they write. Each book in the series contains chapters, called Hacks, composed of these sections:

- **The Problem:** Something you are currently wrestling with that doesn't yet have a clear-cut solution.

- **The Hack:** A brief description of the author's prescribed solution.

- **What You Can Do Tomorrow:** Ways you can take the Hack, or strategy, and implement it right away. These are practical, do-now strategies that readers can use immediately.

- **Building Momentum:** A step-by-step system for turning the do-nows into long-term habits.

- **Removing Obstacles:** A list of possible hurdles you might encounter in your attempt to implement the Hack, and how to overcome them.

- **The Hack in Action:** A snapshot of someone who uses this Hack in their space and how they do it.

OUR PROMISE

Every Hack Learning Life book provides insight, imagination, engaging prose, practical advice, and a little humor. When you read a Hack Learning Life book, you'll have solutions you didn't have before, and when you put our Hacks into action, your daily life will be better for it.

STARTING (AGAIN)

The first moments count more than the later ones.
— DAN CHARNAS, AUTHOR OF *WORK CLEAN*

HOW YOU START matters more than how you finish because you can't finish what you don't start. You can also start so badly that you completely lose control over the quality of the finish. My purpose in writing this book is to help you start (or restart) well by finding simple strategies to create and celebrate small wins along your health journey. If the goal is sustainable health, then the steps you take to get there need to be sustainable as well.

If your "good choices" are working for you only because of your present condition, how long do you think they will last when your conditions change? Making quality food choices, being kind to yourself, choosing consistent movement over being sedentary, finding healthy outlets to deal with and minimize stress, prioritizing sleep, and investing in positive relationships cannot be determined by your circumstances. If you wait until the time is right, until life is easier or the stars align, to make your health a priority, then you will wake up one day and wonder how your health slipped by you. If you have the opportunity to change any (or all) of these factors now, then change them NOW. There will be a day when either the opportunity, ability, or desire to change has passed you by.

In our world, poor options are too often the easiest choice. Candy on the counter. Drive-thru in a rush. Alcohol to ease the tension. Phone scrolling when you're bored. Letting "one more episode" keep you up half the night binge-watching a favorite show. A little lie to alleviate your sense of responsibility for your health. We are good at making destructive habits easy and constructive habits hard. This book is all about how you can make better choices that create small wins and add up to big health.

You are not broken. Your body is a living marvel. You already have some good habits in your life. You just need to expand them to your problem areas. If you keep making the same choices and putting yourself in the same situations with no strategy, then you will likely keep choosing what's easy right now. And we both know where that leads. Where are you struggling right now? You don't have to stay there. You can't afford to stay there.

It is tempting to view our health from a deficit mindset. When I get stressed, caught up in the mundane and wanting to see instant results, I fall into the trap of assuming that what I can see in the moment is all that exists. The narrative ends up being, "This isn't working. There's no way out. I guess this is just how things will be from here on out." I wouldn't ever say those phrases out loud because I know that would sound ridiculous, but my attitude and actions demonstrate that sense of despondency.

The reality of our lives is that the world is an extremely abundant place. An infinite variety of paths lead to a healthier and happier you. But the consumer culture, the outrage culture, the cash grab culture, the instant gratification culture, the news-is-money culture, and the comparison culture of social media all combine to make that abundance challenging to see. Everyone wants to sell you their specific path to help you feel more fulfilled in life. I'm here to tell you that you don't have to buy into a one-size-fits-all approach to health. I want you to experience the joy of building the healthier version of you through better habits, more knowledge, and choices that make you feel proud every day.

My hope here is not to lay out a generic program for health. My goal is to lay a groundwork of unquestionable nutrition, exercise, and mindset principles paired with proven, practical, and actionable steps. The principles without the practical are useless. And the practical without the principles won't carry sufficient impact. It won't surprise you to learn that health topics are quite contentious in today's public forum. Correcting societal issues of food deserts, obesity, weight loss, body composition, healthcare, medications, family upbringing, and cultural norms are beyond the scope of this book. But helping you as an individual and important member of society find a path to more sustainable health is the focal point of this entire work.

I refuse to buy into the deficit mindset. I believe an abundance of people want authentic and genuine healthy social connections. I believe an abundance of people value honesty, encouragement, community, kindness, and self-lessness. I believe we have abundant opportunities to do good, to provide for those who depend on us, to enjoy activity, to honor God with all he has blessed us with, and to have a more abundant life. I am grateful for this opportunity to share my thoughts and journey with you. I will be overjoyed to hear from you one day that something in these words made a difference in your life.

PLAN BIG, WIN SMALL
Unlock the Path to Big Results with Daily Wins

*There are many ways of going forward,
but only one way of standing still.*
— FRANKLIN D. ROOSEVELT, FORMER US PRESIDENT

THE PROBLEM: WE MISS THE SMALL WINS WHEN WE ONLY LOOK FOR BIG RESULTS

HAVE YOU EVER started strong on a new health routine and then dropped off due to frustration? You are not alone. When we examine the challenges that face us in improving our health and well-being, the greatest hurdle is a lack of consistency in exercise and diet. This lack of consistency is often explained away by using excuses like: "I don't have time," "I'm too stressed," "I don't know where to start," "Exercise is boring," "Eating healthy is too confusing," "I'll start Monday," or my personal favorite, "I'm just not motivated." We know we need consistency to see progress in our health journey, so we are driven to find justification for why we are so inconsistent.

Change feels hard. Our brains are wired for safety and happiness. Initiating a change to our current habits can feel unsafe or like a disruption to our happiness, causing our brains to react out of a desire to protect what we have normalized. But what if stagnation is what is holding us back from experiencing more from life? What if staying where we are is the most dangerous place to be? Change is necessary, but it doesn't have to feel daunting.

When you leave something to chance, you are choosing to make it more difficult than it needs to be. Guessing and leaving situations open-ended makes change feel scarier. For example, saying things like "I am going to eat cleaner" is open-ended and leaves too much to chance. Cleaner holds entirely different meanings to different people. It also holds different meanings in different situations. Eating cleaner to one person might be completely cutting out entire food groups, but to another person, it might mean not eating fast food. The definition is too broad to be of use unless you define it carefully. In-the-moment decision-making to find "cleaner" options will quickly lead to feeling over-whelmed and frustrated. What follows from there is usually a return to old eating patterns and a sense of guilt for not following through on the broad goal of eating cleaner. The change was too big and too vague.

Many adults have doubts and fears about sticking to an exercise program, signing up for a gym membership, or committing to a nutrition plan. In some cases, these concerns are valid, but in most instances, creating a pattern of small, attainable wins would greatly assist in diminishing the primary causes of concern. The changes feel too hard, so our brain invents a plethora of justifications for not even trying.

Those excuses, and others like them, do not get to the root of why we so often lack consistency when it comes to making healthy choices in our lives. The true root stems from two often unrealistic assumptions: 1) assuming that the actions ahead will be too challenging or difficult to complete, and 2) assuming that, once started, these actions will achieve immediate major results. We tend to exaggerate how difficult transformation will be and how painful our new choices will feel. Picture what a healthy diet looks like for a moment. Do you imagine bland baked chicken, steamed broccoli, and only water to drink? A lot of people do. Now imagine a weekly exercise routine. Do you picture thousands of crunches, hours of cardio, and mindless repetitions, seven days a week? To many people, this is what comes to mind. No wonder so many are turned off by anything labeled "healthy." We create a false, overinflated picture of what the task will look like to avoid even starting.

Along with overestimating how difficult a healthy lifestyle will be, the second assumption is that if we finally give in to completing those grueling tasks, massive results will naturally follow quickly. Much of the fitness and diet marketing pushed at the general population feeds this mindset with promises of quick results, rapid weight loss, or instant fixes. The all-or-nothing model will not work here (more about that in Hack 10). It is remarkably easy to lose motivation by making a multitude of drastic changes all at once with unreasonable expectations. Too much, too fast, is far more of a hindrance than a help. Overcoming these two hurdles to sustainable actions and consistency is vital in making long-term health and wellness changes.

THE HACK: PLAN BIG, WIN SMALL

The most important piece to building new skills and seeing progress is consistent practice. We know this intuitively and through observation of the world around us. No one becomes proficient at a field of study, hobby, skill set, or knowledge set without consistently applying themselves to the tasks of that craft. The same applies to creating good health. One amazing fact about your brain is that it can quickly adapt to reward new actions and see them as stimulators of happiness. You can build and stack small wins to make change enjoyable, but this takes planning so you can stay in the game long enough to build the skills you need.

Planning future actions and making decisions ahead of time reduces uncertainty and decision fatigue. The lack of planning around the goal of eating "cleaner" is a clear example. The alternative to that vague decision is to plan out a few high-quality food options that you feel good about ahead of time. Instead of a sugary cereal for breakfast, you could plan to have a cup of plain Greek yogurt with fresh fruit. The same goes for movement. Instead of sitting on the couch during an episode of your favorite show, sit on the floor and do some light yoga or stretching while you watch. This will go a long way in reducing the likelihood of that downward spiral of frustration and disappointment, and it will make sticking to your goal so much more sustainable. Make the decision in advance, and be specific about how you will follow through.

Once you have some simple planning in place, it is so much easier to identify the small wins. Small wins are the key to sustainable actions. Small wins create momentum and teach your brain that these new actions are worthwhile and should be rewarded. Consistently showing up won't be likely if you don't see results in the actions themselves and feel rewarded for doing them. Small daily wins teach your brain to reinforce what led to the win. Build the small wins into your regular routine, and you will see how simple those actions feel after a bit of practice.

Let's go back to our example of eating cleaner. Finding small wins in eating a more balanced diet using the foods you prepared or planned will speed up the process of adjusting to this new habit. Celebrating that small victory day after day will ingrain this new habit and make it more enjoyable to stick to. Only you get to decide what is worth celebrating. A win is a win, no matter how small, and we can actively choose to celebrate each one. Notice when you follow through on your decisions. Highlight the feeling you have when you stick to your plan so that your brain remembers how it feels to follow through.

A successful pattern of wins will start with planning and get stronger with practice. This works for exercise just as it works for nutrition. Maybe you are struggling to get started with an exercise program. Start with your plan. The plan should include 1) a space that feels the least restrictive as possible, 2) a clear starting objective that can be accomplished in the first five to ten minutes of the workout, and 3) a mindset focused on your why. With those three planning pieces in place, practice becomes so much easier. Then list out three to five small, daily goals you can aim for to start winning small. Planning the big picture but focusing on the small wins is the best way to build sustainable health habits that can stick with you for life!

WHAT YOU CAN DO TOMORROW

- **Plan two nonnegotiables.** What are two healthy actions that you can realistically complete tomorrow? These need to be doable in a limited time frame but also have a direct impact on your well-being. Once you have them, write them down and schedule them on your calendar. Maybe this is a fifteen-to-twenty-minute walk. Maybe this is a home-cooked meal instead of hitting the drive-thru. Don't leave these actions up to chance or try to "squeeze them in." Nonnegotiables are essential priorities that deserve a designated space in your schedule. These actions will likely end up becoming staples of your health routine and self-care, so don't take this step for granted.

- **Identify two or three small wins to look for tomorrow.** What are two or three actions that you know you can complete tomorrow and that you will feel good about accomplishing? These can be the same as your nonnegotiables, or they can be more bite-sized targets. Maybe you set a step-count goal for the day. Or you decide to replace one highly processed snack with a better-quality snack. These do not have to be difficult, but they need to be clear actions you can check off. If you aren't looking for wins, you probably won't notice them.

- **Start a daily win log.** Sometimes noticing isn't enough for our brains to hold on to. Daily journaling is an incredible mindfulness tool, and including daily wins in a journaling habit is a powerful add-on. But for someone without a journaling habit, a daily win log by itself is an incredible starting point. Focusing on the positive choices you made or the daily targets you accomplished will help give you a positive outlook and make consistency more fun. Another enjoyable aspect of win logs is being able to look back at wins you were celebrating months ago and see how much you've grown.

- **Celebrate small wins.** Celebrating small wins is key to overcoming the fear of failure and self-doubt. You will see more of whatever you focus on ... the defeats, the struggles, or the wins. Celebrate showing up. Celebrate hitting your workout objective. Celebrate adding one or two new challenges each week or month. Celebrate trial and error. How you celebrate is up to you. Do you remember getting stickers on your work in elementary school? It felt good to earn a sticker, even knowing that it had no monetary or intrinsic value. The reward was both tangible and emotional. What are your "stickers" as an adult? Can you find visible or emotional ways to celebrate small wins? It often doesn't take much to reward your brain. Plus, you can find ways to celebrate that align with your personal goals (like visiting a new national park as a celebration of hitting your movement goals for the month) and keep the momentum rolling. Win-win!

BUILDING MOMENTUM

We've all seen a child completely unfazed by their parent's warnings. The child most likely learned that there would not be any follow-up or consequences to those warnings. Your mind is like that child; it's listening to your thoughts much of the time. Real change will start when your mind learns that you will follow through on what you say. Your brain craves patterns and consistency. It is easy to say what should happen or what actions you need to accomplish, but without follow-through, it is just noise. Momentum requires a shift away from saying what we should do for our health to actually getting it done. Building momentum in your health journey through small wins requires changing your habits and mindset in sustainable ways.

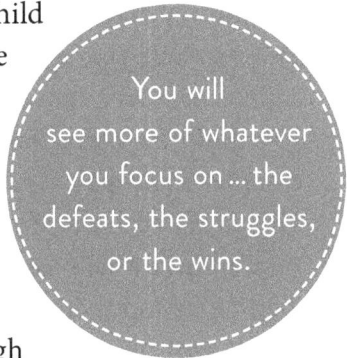

> You will see more of whatever you focus on ... the defeats, the struggles, or the wins.

The power of small wins is found in the reinforcement of daily decisions that compound over time into life-changing and lasting habits. Creating a pattern of small wins starts with daily decisions you can stick to, carries over into how you set concrete goals, and culminates in how you reward and reinforce your new choices. These three steps will guide you through the process of changing 1) what you do, 2) how you follow through, and 3) why you'll stick it out.

STEP 1: Stack habits.

Find simple habits you are already doing well. These are healthy routines that are already ingrained and working well for you. You do not feel decision fatigue about these actions or worry about losing motivation to do them. Now you build on them. Find a new action that you want to complete, and pair it with one of your established habits. This is called habit stacking. Habit stacking reduces friction around a new action by associating it in your brain with an action that already feels easy. Over time, that new action will be second nature in the same way that your original habit already felt frictionless.

A great example is to add (or stack) preparing your exercise clothes or packing your gym bag as part of your bedtime routine. You already have a bedtime routine for changing into your pj's, brushing your teeth, and washing your face. You are preparing to sleep well, so it is a great opportunity to prepare to wake up well. Have the items you need to make your health goals a reality prepared before you go to bed. You can greatly reduce decision fatigue and unnecessary stress early in your day when you have already done the legwork.

During my final year as a teacher, this strategy was essential for me to get my workouts in. I was teaching high school social studies, was in the first year of my online coaching business, and was a dad of three boys. The only opportunity for me to get my workout in was before school each morning. Before getting ready for bed each night, I packed my work clothes, shower essentials, and meals for the next day, plus set out my workout clothes. Was I tempted to hit snooze when my alarm went off at 4:45 each morning? Heck yeah! But I knew the preparation I had already put in would be wasted if I slept in. It was mentally tougher to unpack my work clothes than to follow through with what I had planned. I was able to integrate next-day preparation into my normal rhythm by adding it to my bedtime preparation, and it made my early morning workouts far more sustainable for me.

STEP 2: **Speak your implementation intentions.**

Eliminate "I should" statements from your vocabulary. You are creating ongoing cognitive dissonance, or what I often call mental noise, daily when you say you should do this or that but then don't follow through. Saying one thing and doing another reinforces feelings of inadequacy, mental frustration, and loss of positive momentum. You can replace "I should" statements with implementation intentions.

In basic terms, implementation intentions attach a desired action to a sequence or pattern of events. For example, instead of saying, "I should go to the gym today," you say, "When I leave work, I *will* drive straight to the gym." You have taken a vague, nondescript desired action and connected it to a triggering action. A triggering action is an action that easily carries over to or from another action. Over time, this trigger will become routine and you will have built a new mental pattern. It doesn't matter if the triggering action comes before or after the desired action. Let's say you want to drink more water during the day. An implementation you could use might be: "Before I have a cup

SMALL WINS, BIG HEALTH

of coffee, I will drink a glass of water." Our brains thrive on patterns, so much so that our brains create patterns even when events are entirely random. Implementation intentions help us create patterns purposefully.

Catch yourself when you say "I should" statements. Write them down. Now convert them into implementation intentions. "I should go for a walk today" becomes "I will go for a fifteen-minute walk immediately after dinner." Set these intentions in place in advance—the night before, the week before. Any time frame works as long as it is not "in the moment." Follow through with your statements, and you will develop consistency in completing desired actions and not just hoping you get to them sometime.

I have always been a snacker. I love to graze and munch throughout the day. I used to do this mindlessly, but by using implementation intentions, I am much more mindful and purposeful in how I snack. My favorite statement I use around snacking is: "Before I snack, I will eat a high-quality protein source." The results have been remarkable in that: 1) I am that much closer to hitting my daily protein targets, and 2) I am much less likely to over-snack or make poor snack choices when I am already satiated from the protein. By using a positive triggering action, I can influence the quality of my other decisions.

STEP 3: Create reward structures.

Ever thought about how casinos keep people coming back time after time? The science behind the gambling phenomenon is built on hacking your brain's reward structures. Near wins, occasional wins, sounds, the atmosphere, and a sense of community are just some of the ways casinos reinforce gambling frequency. Gamblers are not motivated in the traditional sense of the word. They are hopeful of a future return.

Positive momentum toward better health is easily sabotaged in the absence of reinforcement. The right choices can often start to feel mundane, or results seem slow to show up. Creating appropriate reward structures will ensure you maintain momentum because you have a sense of hopeful expectancy for what's next.

Find smaller targets to set and celebrate. Humans are not naturally great at delayed gratification. Instead of setting a larger goal to lose ten pounds, set up incremental targets of two pounds at a time. Waiting to celebrate only after losing ten pounds is too delayed. By celebrating every two pounds, you will increase the frequency of celebrating a win by five times! Building a structure of incremental targets will work for strength-gaining programs, running split times, and even daily nutrition targets.

Experiment with rewards that keep you feeling empowered. Rewards can be as simple as noticing what you did (see the daily win log idea discussed earlier) or as complex as a celebration event or trip. You know yourself better than anyone. What makes you feel a sense of fulfillment or excitement? This is a self-designed reward system, so you get to determine what rewards to pair with what accomplishments. You will see more of what you focus on, so focus on your wins and have fun with your rewards.

When I find myself refusing to act on a habit I know is best for me, I remind myself what it felt like the last time

I "won" from that action. Remembering that last workout where I felt so much stress relief is enough to trigger my brain to get moving again. I have a playlist I only listen to when I am walking. I plan quarterly solo hikes to reward myself for the hours I put into my business and to plan out future steps. I share exciting updates with my wife and close circle for social support. Rewards are not selfish. They are essential to growth and pursuing the future of our dreams.

REMOVING OBSTACLES

You might feel reluctant to put action to these ideas. That's normal when facing potential changes. Here are a few common concerns and how you can address them.

I don't have the self-discipline. Self-discipline is essentially keeping your word to yourself. If you feel like you lack discipline, it is likely that you are saying too much to yourself or setting unrealistic expectations. Lower the stakes. Discipline is a learned skill that takes time to build up. If you are reading this book, you have self-discipline in at least a few areas of your life. Examine where your self-discipline came from and what compounding actions helped you build up that skill set. Skills are transferable, so you can take those steps and apply them to your health journey too.

I feel overwhelmed with how much I need to change. Action supersedes fear. Tasks often feel daunting until we get into them and realize our dread was misplaced or exaggerated. Set a five-minute timer and just act. Compartmentalize the different areas that you need to change and focus on small wins in one area at a time. As you build momentum and stack new habits, your capacity to change will increase.

I don't have time to plan. Start with just fifteen minutes, two times a week. Planning can seem like a big ordeal, but it doesn't have to be. Your first fifteen-minute planning time is to set your nonnegotiables (i.e., the habits you are *not* willing to let go of). Your second fifteen-minute planning time is to eliminate nonessentials (i.e., the habits you *are* willing to let go of). Schedule your nonnegotiables and declutter the non-essentials. Start there, and you will be well on your way to a better health plan (more on this in Hack 2).

I struggle to find rewards that work. The best starting point is with the activities you naturally want to do outside of your responsibilities or those you already enjoy but that you can save specifically as a reward. Think through free activities you like, entertainment options that are fun, self-care activities you look forward to, and travel/outdoor pursuits. These can be recurring or one-off rewards. I enjoy trying different pens. So, a reward that would work for me is when I am consistent with my daily win log for a full week, I will get a new pen to try. Or when I am making a healthy meal, I will watch a YouTube channel I enjoy. Don't overthink it. Have fun designing your reward structure, and you'll enjoy your new routines more than ever.

THE HACK IN ACTION

Kevin had zero interest in joining a gym. He told me gyms made him self-conscious, and it was overwhelming to think about exercising around other people. So, I created an at-home workout program for him, and we got to work building up his confidence and new habits.

Two months later, I got a selfie from Kevin of him and his wife at a gym after working out together. Here is what Kevin told me: "My win this month was to make the leap and have the courage to join a gym. Another win was having people mention that I seemed to have gained a new confidence in myself!" I was so excited and proud to see Kevin make this jump, not because you have to join a gym to be healthy but because he was done letting his fears define him. What steps did we take over those two months that helped him build small wins and gain this level of self-confidence?

Kevin had a daily win log that lasted for three weeks. He recorded one to two small wins each day that made him proud of his efforts or actions. He shared these with me at the end of every week so I could support him and encourage him to continue. Week to week, he celebrated better food choices, more activity, more confidence with weights, and more of a desire to push himself.

He also had a weekly workout program that focused on building slowly with good form and mastering each movement. Over the course of two training cycles, Kevin was already pushing his capacity beyond the weights and equipment he had available at home. By focusing on what he could do now, we could get him to a higher threshold and create a desire to see more wins with each workout.

Oddly enough, joining a gym acted as a reward at this point in Kevin's journey. The action he said he didn't want to take became a point of pride and accomplishment for him. Kevin wanted to be able to push himself harder and work out together with his wife, so joining a gym made sense. We spent a few months building up his confidence even more with weights and machines until we reached a point where Kevin was telling me stories of how he was helping other gym-goers with machines and offering tips.

Six months into his journey, Kevin was relying on his gym workouts as a major outlet for both stress relief and self-discipline. He was hitting personal targets each month, had a strong pattern of consistent wins, and was well on his way toward his weight-loss goals. Lasting change takes a combination of planning well and winning small. It didn't always feel easy, and there were tough weeks in Kevin's story, but he would tell you that all the challenges were entirely worth the results.

Fixating on big results is a surefire way to miss ever seeing them. Expecting that change will be difficult will keep you from starting down a new path. But you are in charge of the goals you set, and you are in control of the wins you'll see. When you develop the skill of planning more and winning smaller, you will feel more empowered and capable of finding lasting transformational change. *How* you start matters more in the initial stages than *what* you start. Starting smart, small, and slow might feel "off," but you will build a pattern of success that your brain and body will reward for the long term.

RECLAIM YOUR TIME

Make Your Health a Priority
Even When Time Is Short

*It will never rain roses: when we want to have
more roses, we must plant more roses.*
— GEORGE ELIOT, NOVELIST

THE PROBLEM: WE THINK HEALTHY
ONLY HAPPENS IN OUR FREE TIME

EVERYWHERE WE LOOK, we can find apps and content that promise to "save you time." Any information we need is at our fingertips instantly. Any item we want is only a click away and will be delivered to us in record time. But despite all these technological advancements of convenience, connectivity, and opportunity, the feeling of time scarcity seems to grow daily. The thought of adding more to our plate, even if it's for the sake of our health, feels like a luxury we can't afford or another draining time crunch.

The consequences of feeling time-strapped are significant. It can lead to increased anxiety, chronic stress, and an overall decline in mental and physical well-being. Physical health is directly impacted when we neglect self-care activities such as daily exercise, balanced nutrition, and quality sleep. Relationships also suffer as quality time with loved ones diminishes, resulting in further feelings of isolation and social detachment.

I talk to people weekly who do not make positive steps toward their health because they feel they don't have enough time. Their reasons typically fall into one to four categories: 1) Time for health goals is seen as a luxury. 2) Time for health goals is seen as a task to add on top of a full schedule. 3) Time for health goals is seen as secondary to work and family life. 4) Time for health goals is seen as optional.

Each of these four categories has a ring of truth to it. But the most powerful lies always do. When you believe that time is your biggest hurdle, when your life is so fast-paced that you can't seem to catch your breath, that is when you are most susceptible to sales tactics that tout easy and instant results. These offers are guaranteed to leave your bank account in worse shape without addressing the root causes of why you gravitated to them in the first place.

Time-saving technology, fast-result gimmicks, and excuses about the lack of free time will never be effective solutions to feeling like you don't have time for your health. You will never have enough time to do everything you want. Marketing firms spend billions of dollars each year to steal your attention because they know the value of your precious time and attention.

Fitness influencers love to tell you that we all have the same twenty-four hours in a day. You and I both know this is a nonsensical statement. Work, family, responsibilities, life experiences, and circumstances are different for everyone and put different constraints on our time. Statements like this and the programs built off them try to induce you into action based on shame and guilt. The truth is that your time is not the same as anyone else's, so your solutions need to look different than what works for other people. The catch is how to prioritize health even when time is the issue.

Integrating healthy choices into the day is a simple process that requires purposeful and practical shifts in our daily actions.

THE HACK: RECLAIM YOUR TIME

The solution to making time for your health won't be found in catchy marketing but rather in your ability to reclaim time to make your health goals a priority. The process of reclaiming time requires two shifts: 1) a mindset shift around what health-conscious decisions look like, and 2) a practical shift in how to integrate your health into your normal day-to-day flow.

A mindset shift about what healthy decisions look like is vital. In Hack 1, we discussed how we tend to exaggerate the difficulty of making good health choices. This is relevant to how we struggle to think about dedicating a significant amount of our precious time to grueling health tasks. I have heard "I'm just too busy to add another thing" from potential clients more times than I can count. The essential problem is that we think of health decisions as being "added" to our full calendars. We need to reframe positive health choices as simple essentials that are at the foundation of our daily habits. We don't add healthy choices; we integrate them.

Integrating healthy choices into the day is a simple process that requires purposeful and practical shifts in our daily actions. This is another opportunity to implement habit stacking. Remember that habit stacking is taking a simple task that you would like to begin doing and pairing it with another habit you have already developed. When we use this process for our fitness goals, I call it "health stacking." You can find simple and time-efficient ways to combine quality health choices into your usual routines. Let's say you have a goal to drink more water during the day. A simple strategy is to fill up a water bottle at night as part of your bedtime routine (we'll do a deep dive into bedtime routines in Hack 5). Place that water bottle on your nightstand. In the morning, you will have a visual reminder to drink that water before anything else. You can also stack on the habit of not checking your phone until that bottle is empty, giving you another opportunity for mindfulness as you start your day. This will take no extra time out of your day, and it moves you closer to your daily goal.

Another example of integrating health choices into the day, or health stacking, is to wear comfortable walking shoes when you're on the go. If you are wearing uncomfortable shoes, you might bypass opportunities to increase your daily step count, and you might have sore feet, making you less enthusiastic about completing a workout. Use comfortable walking shoes as a trigger to get in extra steps by parking further away, taking the stairs, moving around while on phone calls, scheduling walking meetings, and stretching when on hold or taking a quick work break. You won't feel like these actions are consuming time because you're stacking the extra movement on top of your preexisting routines.

The healthier version of you probably won't spend hours more per day exercising or preparing food than you currently spend. The healthier version of you probably won't have less demands on your time or a greater abundance of free time. The healthier version of you will be more efficient with the time you have and make more health-conscious decisions during the day. And the healthier version of you won't wait until you "have time" for your health.

As a business owner, trainer, and dad of four boys, I have a lot of demands on my time. Yet, I typically do not feel mental friction around consistently making daily positive health decisions. My normal, my default, is filled with decisions that keep my health goals front and center. And most of those decisions are now subconscious, and I do not feel like they take time away from my work or family priorities. For me, that looks like taking family walks, packing healthy snacks for the next day during kitchen cleanup, drinking water with meals, syncing calendars and meal planning with my wife, setting screen-time limits, and doing light stretching during mental breaks from work.

WHAT YOU CAN DO TOMORROW

- **Set a firm bedtime.** How much sleep do you need to function at your best? What time do you need to wake up? Count back the hours from your alarm and set a firm bedtime that will allow you to get the hours of sleep you need. Don't think of sleep as less time to get things done. Think of sleep as a time quality booster. The more consistent you are with a set bedtime, the more mental and physical energy you will gain. More quality sleep equals a more effective use of your waking hours.

- **Put the phone down.** If you are like most people, the draw of your phone is the biggest time waster in your daily life. Whether it is mindless scrolling or work emails, having a constant connection to the broader world does not positively impact our mental or physical health. Spend less time on comparison and more on preparation. Spend less time consuming and more time producing. Do something fun and leave the phone behind. Stay off devices at night. Set screen limits as time boundaries. Your health is more important than that video or message.

- **Plan the night before.** I can't emphasize this enough: Your brain is not wired to plan when you first wake up. You are most likely not fully alert, fully focused, or ready to make a slew of important decisions. How you wake up sets the tone for your day. Would you rather wake up trying to "wing it" or wake up unperturbed because the morning logistics are already covered? Have your clothes ready. Have breakfast ready or planned. Know what's on your calendar for the day. Do whatever makes sense for you to start your day stress-free rather than jump on the stress carousel.

- **Keep junk foods out of sight.** You probably don't lack impulse control around junk foods. What you lack is an awareness of how junk foods are purposefully designed to hack your brain chemistry. Even the branding, packaging, and taste duration are carefully crafted to stimulate overconsumption. If you leave a jar of candy on your counter and pass by it forty times a day, you will grab a piece at least a few times. It's not impulse control; it's overexposure. Placing that same jar in a drawer will go a long way toward reducing exposure and impulse. Out of sight, out of mind applies to your pantry and fridge as well. Imagine you are tired, stressed, and hungry. If the first thing you see when you open the pantry is brightly colored, easily accessible, high-processed foods, it is unlikely you'll bypass them to prepare a healthier option. Place less-processed foods in more visible locations in your fridge and pantry for an easier time navigating junk food.

BUILDING MOMENTUM

Have you moved to a different home after living in the same house for years or done a big spring cleaning for a yard sale? If you have, you remember being shocked by how much junk you had accumulated without realizing it. Reclaiming and repurposing your time will feel similar. It may be challenging and overwhelming at first, but remember the long-term goal: reducing friction around healthier options for you. With that goal in mind and with a focus on sustainable momentum, you can work on a few simple changes simultaneously regarding how you spend your time—behaviors you clear out of your routine and new behaviors you build into your routine. These strategies will help guide you into 1) a doable weekly fitness routine, 2) a template for planning and editing what consumes your time, and 3) a simple set of questions to help you identify your current priorities. Visit holyfitcoaching.com/smallwins to download free resources, including one to help you reclaim your time.

STEP 1: **Design a three-hour fitness plan.**

Your weekly fitness plan doesn't need to be a part-time job! Ten hours a week is a large amount of time for busy parents, working professionals, and those who travel. You want your fitness routine to be both efficient and attainable. Even if you are only able to dedicate three hours per week to your fitness, you can fit in a lot with the right planning. Each week holds 168 hours. Three hours is 1.7 percent of your week. I believe that is a doable time target for everyone who is willing to try. Here is a simple breakdown of how to spend those hours.

First, block off two distraction-free, fifteen-minute planning times. This is essential. Without planning, you will not sustain healthier habits or eating. The first fifteen-minute block is to plan out your time for workouts, walking, and meal preparation. The items you plan during this period are your nonnegotiables. During the second fifteen-minute block (this can be later in the same day or a different day), you will edit out the nonessentials. It's not enough to know your priorities. You also need to edit out the actions that get in the way of your priorities!

Next up is three thirty-minute workouts per week. I encourage strength training, but any exercise that uses some form of resistance is the most effective way to protect your joints, bones, lean muscle tissue, and mobility. The most efficient use of your time will include a well-structured full-body circuit. This includes a warm-up and some combination of the primary body movements of push, pull, squat, lunge, and hinge. We live in the golden age of access to workouts. App-based training, YouTube workouts, and group fitness options are plentiful. You can also have personalized workouts created for you by a fitness trainer. Options abound; what's most important is your consistency.

The next step is to set aside one hour for meal prep. Meal prep can feel scary, but it doesn't need to be. One hour is enough time to prepare a few balanced and nutritious meals for the week. I coach all my clients to plan their most challenging meals first. If eating a quality breakfast is a struggle, start by packing three great breakfasts in advance that you can grab during the week. If your nutrition choices are a struggle on Thursdays and Fridays, then prepare and freeze your lunches for those two days over the prior weekend when you have more time to plan ahead. Don't overcomplicate this at the start. Simple and effective meal prep will get you on a great trajectory you can build on later.

The final step is to increase your NEAT time. NEAT stands for non-exercise activity thermogenesis, which basically means daily energy output that is in addition to purposeful exercise. Leisurely walks, taking the stairs, casual outdoor activities, and yard work are examples of movement classified as NEAT. For most people, accumulating 120 to 180 minutes a week is a great range of daily activity levels. This time is not built into your three-hour fitness plan but is integrated into your usual daily activities. Aim to include types of movement you enjoy and can do regularly. You are making sustainable health easier when you increase your daily activity, purposeful exercise, and planning times.

STEP 2: **Deploy a three-stage planning and editing timeline.**

Planning and editing your priorities can be a daunting task without a clear roadmap. In Hack 1, we talked about eliminating "I should" statements. Lasting change comes from grounded and doable actions based on attainable hopes, not just from lofty goals. Let's dive deeper into the practical steps of planning and editing your week-to-week activities.

First, list your three primary action priorities. These are *not* your goals or the results you hope to achieve. These should be clear actions you will take for your health daily or, at a minimum, several times per week. Write them down in the format of "I will do x," "I will make y," or "I will take z." A great example is "I will take a thirty-minute walk."

Now it's time to schedule your action priorities. Plan them. Make them nonnegotiables. Nonnegotiable means that as much as it is in your power, you will hold yourself to completing these actions. Take your existing "I will do x" statements and add a day and time. Going back to our walking example, you might decide that Tuesday, Thursday, and Saturday mornings work best for your schedule. Your statement then becomes "I will take a thirty-minute walk on Tuesday, Thursday, and Saturday mornings."

The final step in your planning timeline is to cut out the nonessentials that interfere. Most of the friction we face is in the form of preexisting habits or mental clutter. These are clearly items you can and should let go of. What *habits* do you have now that will make your new priority actions more challenging to complete? You'll either need to limit them or cut them out entirely. What *thoughts* do you have now that will make your new priority actions more challenging to complete? You edited your schedule, now edit your thoughts. Declutter your mind through meditation, prayer, therapy, or some other means that allows you to reduce the friction in making your planned actions actually happen.

STEP 3: **Make three decisions.**

Even on your busiest days, you make countless decisions that either push you along toward a healthier you or pull you back from progressing. If you can begin to shift more of those decisions into the "push" category, the cumulative effect will pay off over time. Here are three simple decision-making statements I like to work through with my clients to help them begin that shift without getting overwhelmed or overthinking it.

- **Decision One: I am okay with letting go of ...** You have to know what you're okay letting go of, especially in stressful or busy seasons. Here's an example from my life: I need to wake up very early most days of the week to train clients. Adequate sleep is a major priority for me, so I am okay with letting go of watching a sports event in order to get to sleep on time. I can watch the highlights later.

- **Decision Two: I am not okay with letting go of ...** You have to know what you're not okay letting go of, especially when life throws you curveballs on a regular basis. In my case, I am not okay with missing many evenings with my kids after they are home from school. Because of that, I do not train clients in the evening. I would rather have that time with my kids than have extra income or a later wake-up alarm!

- **Decision Three: When it gets tough, I will ...** You need a backup plan, especially when starting new patterns or actions. We will focus on this in more detail in Hack 10. Rock climbers have supporting points so that if they do slip up, they will only fall so far. Most people jump into a fitness or health routine without a fallback for when they inevitably struggle. My fallback for busy seasons is to shorten my workouts or replace them with at-home stretching or resistance band sessions.

REMOVING OBSTACLES

Here are a few common concerns for this Hack and how to address them.

I'm too tired to exercise. How do you expect to have energy to exercise if you do not signal to your body that you need energy? Doing the thing is what gives you the ability to do the thing. Your body is constantly adapting to the signals you send it. Make your body move and then rest intentionally. You might be surprised at how quickly your body adjusts to your new normal.

I don't have any accountability. Accountability will never appear out of thin air. It has to be invited in. Accountability naturally occurs when you place yourself in community with like-minded people who are pursuing similar goals as you. Are you regularly putting yourself into positions that invite accountability? Those positions could be local clubs, formal or informal relationships, or even online coaching settings. Only when you actively seek accountability will you be able to build a support system that keeps you on track.

I'm bad at time management. We were trained to handle other people's time better than we handle our own. Boundaries are our friends. You are most likely fine at time management (holding a job, earning a degree, or organizing a calendar), but you haven't learned to set effective boundaries around your own priorities. Place tighter boundaries around the areas you want to protect most, and you will see your focus and consistency rise.

I don't have the capacity to make an action plan. It's okay if you don't feel confident in your ability to create a plan for yourself, especially when your time is so valuable. I don't feel confident in my ability to do home repairs. I ask for help from folks in my circle or from professionals. If time constraints make your health feel impossible to hold onto, maybe it's a sign to bring someone into your life who has an outside perspective. I can speak from experience about the

Accountability will never appear out of thin air. It has to be invited in.

value of delegating your health program design and time-table to a trusted professional. Don't feel like you have to do it all alone.

THE HACK IN ACTION

Aaron wasn't trying to be super jacked or the world's strongest man. He was tired of being in pain and fearing exercise. He wanted to get back to moving his body to better serve God and his family for a long time. Aaron is a dad of three girls, a passionate leader in a global nonprofit organization, and someone who has been an athlete his entire life. But when his body started to shut down in 2021, he began an uncertain journey of learning to live with Type 1 narcolepsy. After over two years of episodes and fatigue, Aaron had allowed nonstop work, a lack of boundaries, and mental fear about exercise to leave him depleted and not sure how to get his strength back.

Aaron jumped into a six-week dad challenge that I was promoting. He was cautious about getting back into regular exercise but knew that I would ease him back into health and help him rebuild. Aaron was coming off the Christmas season, the busiest season for a Christian non-profit, and decided to start the New Year with a new priority of "leading self." Aware of his time constraints and physical obstacles, we dove into the challenge with a focus on a clear weekly plan and building consistency without trying to pack too much into his day.

Aaron carved out three mornings a week to start his day with exercise. He knew that leading others well meant he had to lead himself well. He called this "leading self" and began to tweak his habits. We had to start small. We got him planning healthier meals with higher protein and being more conscious of food choices when having lunch with donors. We worked on getting his daily steps up and building in movement breaks. Aaron's workout plan wasn't about high intensity or maximum weight. It was about making movement feel doable, completing a workout even when he wasn't feeling his best, and getting his body a bit stronger with weights.

Aaron put in the work. He didn't make excuses, even though it felt hard at first and time was short. He followed the three-hour fitness strategy with three short workouts per week, daily walks, and putting up more boundaries around work. This approach not only fit Aaron's schedule but also delivered incredible results.

Within six weeks, Aaron was stronger and loved being back in the gym. At the end of the program, he messaged me to share his biggest takeaways, writing:

"My initial goal was to get back into the gym, and I've definitely been able to do that. I'm figuring out the areas that I can push my body in again. Competitive sports aren't possible for me and probably never will be again, but the gym has been great! A few big wins for me: 1) I'm back in the gym, 2) I've adjusted my weekly schedule to prioritize my health, and 3) my wife has also been working out/running multiple times a week – lots of pros to that!"

Even in the face of illness, fatigue, and a lack of time, Aaron showed up with unwavering dedication, motivated by the knowledge that every minute invested in himself was a step toward reclaiming the life he wanted to live. The walks, the quick stretching and mobility exercises, simple nutrition changes, weekly scheduling, regular self-reflection, and hydration hacks all fit into his life because he made it work and kept the big picture in mind. Aaron knows his health is a vital part of his larger purpose, and months later, he continues to make it a priority in his busy schedule.

Aaron's story serves as a testament to the power of using time effectively. It also showcases how there will never be a perfect time to start. Even in the face of overwhelming responsibilities, you can find moments for self-care and personal growth. Through intentional choices and a steadfast commitment to his well-being, Aaron pushed through, reminding us that it's never too late to reclaim strength and reframe our priorities.

The excuse of not having enough time seems to let us off the hook. It's like an umbrella we can hide under without taking any steps to get out of the pouring rain. It might shield our egos but doesn't do anything to remedy the far-from-ideal situation we happen to be in. To paraphrase the epithet of this chapter: "Life will never shower you with health: when we want to have more health, we must make use of time to create more health." The lack or abundance of free time is not the deciding factor for your health. You can't make more time, but you can make better use of the time you have. You can use your time in ways that create less friction along the path to a healthier you.

EAT LIKE YOU MEAN IT
Eat On Purpose for Balance and Sustainability

The table is a meeting place, a gathering ground,
the source of sustenance and nourishment,
festivity, safety, and satisfaction.
— LAURIE COLWIN, AUTHOR

THE PROBLEM: WE EAT FOR CONVENIENCE AND COMFORT

IN TODAY'S FAST-PACED society, convenience often takes precedence over proper nutrition, leading to detrimental effects on general health and increasing stress and anxiety surrounding food, what we should and shouldn't eat, and dieting habits.

At the core of the issue is the prevalence of fast food, highly processed meals, and snacks that have become staples in our diets. These foods are often highly palatable and high in unhealthy fats and added sugars while lacking essential nutrients like fiber, vitamins, and minerals.

The convenience-focused culture surrounding food choices also promotes mindless eating and a disconnect from the actual process of nourishing your body. Eating on the go, in front of screens, or in a rushed manner diminishes the enjoyment and mindfulness associated with meals. The convenience of grabbing a quick meal on the go or ordering takeout has led to a significant decline in home-cooked, wholesome meals. Food is an object of fixation and often devoid of the pleasure of being prepared in the home and part of engaging in communal dining experiences.

This overreliance on quick fixes has resulted in a range of negative health impacts. The consumption of highly processed foods contributes to the rising rates of obesity, heart disease, diabetes, and other chronic conditions. These health problems not only affect individuals but also place a significant burden on the healthcare system.

Furthermore, the lack of balance in the American diet has a direct correlation with stress levels. The constant intake of high-sugar, high-fat foods can lead to energy crashes, mood swings, and decreased mental clarity. Along with high stress, overconsumption, and health concerns comes the ever-increasing presence of weight loss marketing and misinformation about healthy approaches to nutrition. Weight loss marketing and the diet culture at large often fall short in addressing the lack of proper nutritional education, how to navigate necessary lifestyle changes, the importance of macronutrients and micronutrients, and individualized metabolic needs. In a society focused on convenience, quick fixes, and the pursuit of an idealized body, diet culture promotes restrictive eating patterns and unrealistic expectations, leading to frustrations and feelings of hopelessness for many who strive to achieve optimal health.

One major issue with diet culture is its tendency to promote fad diets and restrictive eating patterns that often lack scientific evidence and fail to provide adequate nutrition. These diets tend to focus on short-term weight loss goals rather than long-term sustainable health. They often eliminate entire food groups or severely restrict calorie intake, leading to potential nutrient deficiencies, imbalances, or eating disorders.

Moreover, diet culture often overlooks the importance of understanding macronutrients and their role in supporting overall health. While the focus may be on counting calories or eliminating certain foods, the emphasis on macronutrient composition and balance is often neglected. Each macronutrient (carbohydrates, proteins, and fats) plays a crucial role in energy production, hormone regulation, and cellular function. Without some understanding of these macronutrients and their impact on the body, individuals may inadvertently compromise their metabolic needs.

THE HACK: EAT LIKE YOU MEAN IT

Combating the widespread normalization of overconsumption, convenience-focused food culture, and restrictive dieting is a macro-sized problem that can only be addressed at the micro level. It will start with you—with your habits and within your home. Only when you decide enough is enough, take control of what is within your control, and make learning a bit more about nutrition a priority will you find a balanced and sustainable approach to eating mindfully that works for you and your goals.

There is no one-size-fits-all approach to nutrition. There are key principles of nutrition that every individual will benefit from understanding, and there are simple strategies that help make those principles practical to deploy. The ultimate priority is for you to know how to ditch harmful eating habits and gradually replace them with solutions that feel aligned and doable for life. Uncontrolled eating, mindless eating, convenience-focused eating, and overly restrictive eating won't allow you to feel aligned or healthy in the long term. With that common understanding, it's time to dive into core principles of nutrition that are fundamental to a healthy approach to eating.

Food is your source of energy. Some energy sources fuel different aspects of your bodily functions, just like different fluids and oils help a car engine operate effectively. Macronutrients (protein, carbs, and fats) are the three primary categories of energy. Macros are forms of chemical energy, and calories are simply a measure of that energy. A well-balanced diet will include a substantial amount of all three categories of energy. One example of a balanced approach that is manageable for most people is 25 percent protein, 50 percent carbs, and 25 percent fats.

- Proteins are made up of complex chains of essential amino acids. Protein is vital in building all body tissues, including muscle synthesis and hormone and enzyme production. One gram of protein contains a total of 4 calories.

- Carbohydrates also contain 4 calories per gram and are broken down into glucose. Glucose is transported to cells and converted into ATP (adenosine triphosphate) through anaerobic glycolysis.

- Fats contain 9 calories per gram. Fat repels water and is the carrier for the fat-soluble vitamins A, D, E, and K. Fat is another key source of energy through ATP. Our brains are 60 percent fat, and adequate fat intake is necessary for balanced hormone production. We are always burning and always storing fat as adipose tissue to use as energy when required.

Understanding the basics of macronutrients and how the body uses them further illustrates the importance of nutrient-dense foods. If food is fuel, then nutrient-dense foods are better sources of fuel than foods that have been stripped of their nutritional value. Eating mostly nutritionally deficient foods will rob your body of key micronutrients, increase mental and metabolic stress, impede normal digestive functions and gut health, lower your body's immune system and ability to fight inflammation, and increase the potential of many other associated health risks.

Highly processed foods lack the structural and nutritional complexity of whole foods. These foods include what we generally call junk foods but can also include plenty of options that the general public would consider to be "healthier" foods. There are six key markers, or red flags, I teach my clients to look out for in their diets. These markers typically show up in combinations. The higher the number of red flags a food or type of food contains, the more cautious you should be about eating it. The markers are 1) high saturated fat content, 2) high sugar content, 3) high-calorie foods with little nutritional value (check the label for macronutrient and micronutrient info), 4) easier to overeat (not satiating), 5) highly processed, and 6) high flavor stimuli.

Let's dive into simple strategies for swapping foods with these markers for better quality foods that are less processed and more nutritionally rich. A great place to start is to complete a basic food log for three to five days. Simply record everything you consume over this time period without judgment or changing from your existing routine. After completing the food log, you will perform a self-audit. Which foods with multiple red flags show up for you most often? Put these foods into your "red" column. We will dive into this in more detail in the Building Momentum section, but your red-column foods are the ones you need to put more boundaries around to protect your long-term health. This doesn't mean you can never have these foods. It does mean you should focus some energy on finding healthier alternatives as go-to options and save your red-column foods for specific occasions. Visit

If food is fuel, then nutrient-dense foods are better sources of fuel than foods that have been stripped of their nutritional value.

holyfitcoaching.com/smallwins to download free resources, including an ultimate snack guide.

The second major swap is to replace a select number of meals purchased outside the home with ones prepared by you at home. If you consume three or more meals per week from restaurants, fast food, food trucks, or food delivery, you are giving up control of a significant percentage of your meals in terms of portion sizes, quality of ingredients, caloric intake, and impulse control. Even swapping one meal per week is an effective place to start. You can build to a point where dining out is a special occasion or event and not an active part of your lifestyle. Also, begin to emphasize the importance of home-cooked meals over processed and pre-packaged foods. Cooking at home allows you to have control over the ingredients, portion sizes, and cooking methods, ensuring healthier choices and practicing balanced nutrition.

To move away from convenience-focused meals to home-cooked meals, you will need a process for mindful meal planning. Start by creating a weekly meal plan that includes a few staple "go-to" ingredients that can be combined to create a variety of nutritious and balanced meals. Consider the nutritional value, portion sizes, and ingredients when designing your menu. Pick two to three great protein sources, two to three high-quality carb sources, two to three vegetables you enjoy, and two to three healthy fats. For example, a basic shopping list might look like this:

Protein: eggs, chicken breast, lean ground turkey

Carbs: sweet potatoes, brown rice, chickpeas

Vegetables: spinach, carrots, red cabbage

Fats: avocado, extra virgin olive oil, chopped almonds

With these few ingredients, you can mix and match, creating delicious meals to eat at home and to pack for when you are out and about. I love the 3-3-3 model, shown in Image 1, for keeping meals balanced and varied.

3—3—3 STRATEGY

Keep things simple your first few weeks of meal prep. Try the 3-3-3 Method. Choose 3 different protein sources, 3 fat sources, and 3 carb sources only

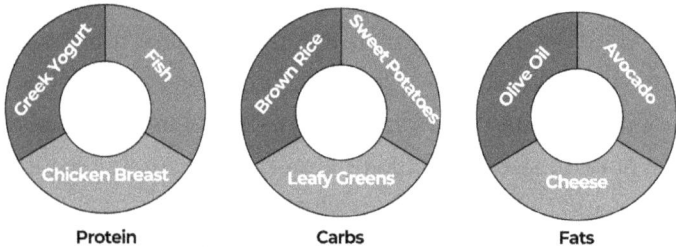

| Protein | Carbs | Fats |

Image 1

Simply identifying your problem foods, swapping restaurant meals for meals at home, and creating a simple meal plan you can actually follow will take you far in becoming more mindful of your eating habits. But you don't have to do this alone. Seek support and inspiration from other people who are committed to the same process, hire a nutrition coach, and join communities or online groups that promote healthy eating habits. Share recipes, meal ideas, and success stories to stay motivated and inspired. Renowned leadership expert John C. Maxwell said, "The better you are at surrounding yourself with people of high potential, the greater your chance for success." Find your community of people who will spur you on, challenge you, and keep you going on those tough days. (For more meal-planning strategies and ideas, check out the "Master Meal Planning" chapter in the book *Hacking Life After 50* by James Alan Sturtevant and Mark Barnes.)

WHAT YOU CAN DO TOMORROW

- **Focus on protein + fiber.** This will reduce cravings and keep blood sugar levels steady. The protein + fiber combo will change the way you eat and snack. You will benefit from more sustained energy, longer fullness signals, better digestion, and more regular bowel movements. You will also keep blood sugar more stable and get off the cravings-to-crash spiral. Greek yogurt + fruit, overnight protein oats, veggies and cottage cheese, no-bake protein power balls (tons of great recipes online), and nuts with cheese are a few great combos to consider.

- **Use hand portion guides.** Portion control is huge. Practice portion control by using smaller plates and bowls to help regulate serving sizes. My favorite method for portion control is to use your hands as your measuring tool. The benefit is that your hands are always with you and remain a consistent size. As a general rule, one palm = a portion of protein, one fist = a portion of vegetables, one cupped hand = a portion of carbs, and one thumb = a portion of fats. Moderately active people will typically have success at creating balanced meals by aiming for one to two portions of each hand size per meal. This strategy comes particularly handy (excuse the pun) when eating at a conference, party, or buffet.

- **Plan a healthy snack.** You will get hungry, and you will be tempted to grab unaligned options when you are on the go. The best strategy is to trust your preparation, not your willpower. Plan healthy snack options in advance. Keep great snacks stocked at work. Invest in a cooler bag for daily cold snacks. Store some shelf-stable options in your car (trail mix, seeds, dried fruit, jerky). Life will surprise you. Control the uncontrollable by having your backup snacks always close by.

- **Eat slower and chew more.** Nutritious food requires more chewing to break down than processed foods. You can experiment with this. Generally, high-processed foods average ten chews per bite by design, whereas whole foods average twenty-five chews. Chewing your food more is an important aspect of the digestion process. Your gut will also thank you if you eat slower. Not only will you give satiety signals time to kick in, but you will also reduce the work-load on your gut. Win-win.

- **Limit liquid calories.** Liquid calories are sneaky. You can easily consume an addi-tional 500 calories per day from liquids alone. High-calorie drinks are highly palat-able, typically contain many added sugars, and don't typically trigger your satiety sig-nals like solid foods. Be mindful about your intake of sweetened beverages and aim for water to be most of your liquid intake.

BUILDING MOMENTUM

Changing long-established eating habits and patterns is no easy feat. Our brains develop deeply rooted patterns quickly that associate taste, texture, and experience with mood-altering chemical responses. Knowing what we should eat and actually doing it are two different things. As a nutrition coach, I spend very little time telling my clients what to eat and a lot more time teaching them the skills of hunger management, coping with stress without food, and helping them find and create new nutrition options that they feel great about. Understanding your default patterns and attachment to certain foods, spotting the triggers of your main problem areas, and finding the small wins as you shift your behavior are the best ways to build momentum toward more mindful eating habits.

STEP 1: **Confront your problem area(s).**

Do you struggle with mindless snacking? The first step is to identify what snacks are easiest for you to overconsume. Maybe this hits you most at night, on weekends, or when you are stressed. There might be different types of snacks under different circumstances, meaning you might not spot all the patterns at once, but if you are paying attention, you will spot them over time. The second step is to replace those problematic snacks with ones that allow you to better control your intake. Today, we have so many easily accessible, delicious, and nutritious snack options available to us.

Do you tend to overeat at meals? Combining the strategies we discussed for eating slower, using the hand portions strategy, and eating balanced meals will help. Another strategy is to focus on consuming your protein source first since protein will produce a higher satiety response than other foods. You will find it difficult to overeat at meals when you slow down, eat larger protein portions, and include grains and vegetables that are high in fiber.

Do you struggle with stress eating? We know that stress reduces both impulse control and fullness signals between your gut and brain. First, determine where the triggers for stress eating are coming from. Second, stop the chain leading to the trigger. We tend to focus on treating the symptoms but ignore the underlying issues. Maybe your lack of quality sleep is keeping your stress levels high (good news: we will dive into sleep habits in Hack 5). Sure, stress eating is a problem. But you need to see that as the visible symptom of deeper pain points.

Do you experience food guilt? I encourage you to drop your "good" and "bad" labels. We tend to label certain foods as good and others as bad, but that is entirely subjective. Using language like better for me, worse for me, eat less, eat some, and eat more can help take the pressure off subjective labels. What you eat is not a question of morals or character. Enjoying food is a human experience and an aspect of life that we can celebrate. Focus on aligned eating (i.e., eat with your goals in mind). When you notice a pattern of unaligned eating, that's when you adjust and plan again.

STEP 2: Follow the 80 percent rule.

No perfect nutrition plan exists. My family doesn't eat 100 percent whole foods 100 percent of the time. Every decision is a tradeoff, and the tradeoff cost of trying to eat a perfect diet is too high. Even professional bodybuilders and elite athletes whose livelihoods depend on their appearance or performance talk about the high levels of mental stress they endure when preparing for peak performance. If they can't do it when it is their full-time job, why do you think you should be able to do it? There is a better way.

I advocate for most people to use the 80 percent rule when they are making their nutrition plan. 80/20 feels doable and easier for us to wrap our heads around. If you ate on plan 80 percent of the time, at three meals a day, you'd have seventeen high-quality, balanced, and aligned meals every week. Compare that to only four meals each week that weren't as high quality. Zoom out, and that would be sixty-eight high-quality meals to sixteen lower-quality meals per month. That ratio, in the long term, would be such an effective pattern of success.

Aim for 80 percent of your intake to be whole foods, and eat until you are 80 percent full. Make your own food 80 percent of the time. The 80 percent rule is all about consistency. This is a much more sustainable approach than the over-restrict/overindulge model that you've probably tried and failed many times before. The more you practice, the easier it gets. And the easier it gets, the more consistent you become. It is far more likely that you will find sustainable health when you have a sustainable diet.

STEP 3: Flag foods as red/yellow/green.

Most of us have foods that we tend to overeat or foods that we might use as a stress response but that make us feel worse in the long term. And then there are the highly processed foods we discussed earlier in the chapter with the combinations of red flags. Foods of these types should go into your "red" category. Red-column foods are ones that you eat less of the time, are easy for you to overeat, or make you feel ill or cause discomfort in any way. Don't feel like you can *never* have them. Simply prioritize higher-quality snacks and treats as your normal go-to options. The "yellow" column is for the foods you are planning to eat some of the time. These are better options—less processed but still not your main go-to options. Foods in your yellow column are for in-a-pinch or on-the-go eating when options are limited or scattered throughout your week. The "green" column is for foods you plan to eat more of and more often. These are foods that align fully with your nutrition goals. Whole-food fats, whole-food carbs, and lean protein sources always get the green light.

The more you practice, the easier it gets. And the easier it gets, the more consistent you become.

REMOVING OBSTACLES

Here are a few common concerns for this Hack and how to address them.

I don't know how to curb my cravings. Cravings are tough. We experience a certain urge, perform a certain behavior, and quickly get a certain reward. And our brains love it. The best way to stop a craving is not through will-power. It is preventing the urge from ever showing up. Many experience intense cravings in the afternoons or evenings. By increasing their protein intake, making sure they eat balanced meals during the workday, and maintaining great snack options, those urges vanish rather quickly. If you can't stop the urge, or a craving randomly shows up, sit with it for five minutes. Just recognize it, identify why it's there, and work through your options. If giving in is the only option, then accept it and move forward. But most of the time, you'll find an alternative that feels more aligned.

My family or home environment isn't supportive. Family and home environments are the biggest factors that most diet approaches never talk about. Changing your eating habits alone or in an unsupportive environment is incredibly challenging. But someone in your family will have to be the one who says, "No more." That person can be you! You can be the one to put an end to generational issues. No one is stopping you from being the change your family needs. Recruit an ally in the home. Teach and involve the family. Search YouTube for videos that show simple, healthy meal options, and watch them together. Encourage willing family members to participate in meal planning, grocery shopping, and cooking to foster a sense of ownership and appreciation for nutritious meals. Launch it with a family cook-off, holiday meal, or monthly "new food" day.

Eating healthy is expensive. It's true that many healthy food options are marketed to and priced for those with more affluent grocery store budgets. But that doesn't mean eating healthy is expensive. Eggs, whole grains, vegetables, canned tuna, sweet potatoes, beans, and peas are a few examples of high-quality food options that are not high priced. Preparing healthy, filling foods in bulk will cost you a lot less money than grabbing fast food, a snack at a convenience store, or pizza.

I get overwhelmed when I think about changing what I eat. This is a completely normal response. Our society puts a lot of pressure around food, and we put a lot of pressure on ourselves to eat perfectly or "clean." The primary goal of any diet change must be: "Can I sustain this in the long term?" If your change is to add 20 grams of protein to your diet each day, is that sustainable? For most people, it is. Or if your goal is to eat one more fist-sized portion of vegetables each day, can you hit that on most days? With some thought put into it, you can. Start where the change feels easiest and most natural. Then it will snowball from there. Ask what you can add to your diet before you think about what to take out. Plenty of poor food choices will automatically fall off if you have enough of the good stuff coming in.

THE HACK IN ACTION

John was twenty-five, and his health was going downhill fast. His parents and siblings had long battled obesity and diabetes. John had always been relatively healthy as a kid, but the impact of his home environment and the stress of running a business while also finishing college to be an educator led him to unhealthy eating habits. John was a hundred pounds overweight and diagnosed as pre-diabetic. He knew he had to make a change.

The biggest change came by way of his eating habits. John had to learn his triggers and not to let stress dictate his choices when it came to food. He wanted to turn to comfort foods on tough days. Limiting and eventually getting rid of those black-and-white cookies (you know which ones I'm talking about) proved to be a long road. But he made the shift over several months and found meals and snacks he could prep from week to week that kept him on track.

John had rough stretches when he went through the yo-yo of focused and unfocused weeks, particularly around the holidays with family or when work stress elevated.

But he knew his triggers, and he also knew that going for walks and having healthy snacks got him past the immediate struggle.

John stopped thinking he had to be perfect to be on track. The 80 percent rule gave him room to be flexible as a working college student and then into his time as a student teacher and long-term substitute teacher.

John sent me a note describing how he had been pushing 270 two years ago and had struggled with a move into his new home due to the effort of carrying items and going up and down the stairs. He had to take breaks because his blood sugar would get too low. He started his health journey just after that move. In the note, he mentioned that he had recently moved again, but this time, "The improvement was remarkable."

John is down seventy pounds, his body fat percentage is in a great spot, and the risk of Type 2 diabetes is way back in the rearview mirror. But most importantly, John is comfortable handling the stress of life because he has confidence in his ability to eat mindfully and find solutions instead of excuses.

⚬⊢⊣⚬

What you eat and how you eat will have a larger cumulative impact on your life than where you work, where you live, what education you have, or the vacations you take. You wouldn't "wing it" when it comes to those important life decisions, so why would you approach what fuels, heals, and protects your body without planning and preparation?

Changing the quality of your food will directly change the quality of your life. You cannot eat perfectly because there is no perfect diet. But you can always eat a little bit better. You can always eat more mindfully, eat foods more aligned with your goals, and do the best you can to care for your body. Don't stress nutrition, but don't neglect it, either. Finding sustainability and balance in your nutrition is a lifelong journey and can include an incredible amount of fun and joy.

MASTER THE MENTAL NOISE
Be a Good Friend to Yourself

You cannot overestimate the unimportance
of practically everything.
— JOHN C. MAXWELL, AUTHOR AND LEADERSHIP EXPERT

THE PROBLEM: OUR THOUGHTS
ARE OUR WORST ENEMY

OFTEN, WHAT WE are thinking about at any given moment feels like the most important thing in the world. But then, as the thought fades, the importance of that thought also fades, only to be brought back into shocking clarity when we think of it again. If we were to journal all our thoughts, we would notice that our thinking tends to cycle around a few central topics most of the time. Most of our thoughts swirl around ourselves: how we perceive ourselves, how we think others perceive us, or how we relate to a situation, object, or choice before us. By default, we become our most important thought, and our perception is shaped and colored by the language of how we think about and talk to ourselves. Our thoughts about ourselves are a jumble of hopes, anxieties, desires, and concerns.

Some might call it self-talk, self-esteem, or our internal dialogue. To me, it's just thinking. It is the way we process, the way we navigate a world too big for us to comprehend. And we don't navigate it very well. The world is bigger than ever, and we are exposed to more of it daily. Not only are we inundated by a constant stream of ideas, but we also are expected to make critical, rapid-fire judgment calls on how we relate to the broader world at every turn. And the infinite comparisons come next. Did I wear the right clothes, say the right words, and respond in the right ways compared to others around me? I don't look as good as them, feel as good as they must, sound as good as they sound, or have the talent they have. The collision of our internal dialogue with the interruption of a big world creates an ever-present noise. Sometimes, it is manageable; other times, it is all we can hear.

If comparison is the thief of joy, then mental noise is the getaway car. Mental noise shows up as fear, reluctance, procrastination, insecurity, indecision, victimhood, or a complaining spirit. Nothing is more anxiety-inducing, fear-producing, or nagging than how we think about ourselves. We create narratives that we tell ourselves over and over. These help us navigate an insane world by creating shortcuts to understanding who we are and what we are about. *I'm this or that, I'm this sign, I fit here, I don't fit there, I'm this type, I could never ..., I will never ....*

These stories serve a limited role but can hold us back from trying new things, taking risks, seeing ourselves in a different light, or true self-reflection.

Most of the friction you face, the reluctance that hinders you from taking a needed step, originates and resides exclusively within your mind. If left unchecked, this mental noise can become your greatest obstacle and the most dangerous form of self-sabotage in your journey to sustainable health.

THE HACK: MASTER THE MENTAL NOISE

Mastering the mental noise begins with a recognition that how we think about ourselves has a tremendous impact on our trajectory. Perception doesn't shape reality, but it does *shade* reality. Imagine for a moment that you are self-conscious about a particular trait or feature you have. You walk around assuming everyone is immediately drawn to that certain aspect of you and that it impacts how they relate to you. I could poll a hundred people who know you well, and the likelihood that anyone would mention that trait or feature is fairly close to zero. Your internal perception is shaping how you show up, independent of what is actually happening outside of your thoughts.

I was always athletic and active. I played multiple sports in high school and soccer in college. I was also skinny. I struggled to eat enough and was underweight for my height, even well into my twenties. I remember going to visit my grandfather and how he grabbed my ribs as he hugged me and joked that I was skin and bones. He was a kind man and meant well, but as a young man, I let that comment stick in my head. I started to become more self-conscious about being thin and thought other people were looking at me through that lens as well. I don't share that story as if it were a traumatic event but more to illustrate an example of a mental thought pattern that I had to work through.

Recognizing that much of your internal self-doubt does not match up with how others see you is a powerful tool. I continued to have self-doubt about my size and strength, particularly when I started working out at a gym. It took me time to work through my insecurities about not being as big as other guys or not being able to lift as much weight. In my case, I allowed how I thought about being weak to keep me from doing the exercises that would get me strong. No one was watching. All of that was just in my head.

Here is the reality: You are the only person stopping you from being healthier. You can blame society, genetics, family history, your astrological sign, or your neighbor's dog that barks all night (okay, that one might be legitimate). But ultimately, you are an adult, and you are responsible for you. You make choices, you build habits, and you spend your money. And every choice you make, habit you build, and dollar you spend could be different if you really wanted it to be. I'm not saying change is easy. But it can be *easier* if you recognize how you are getting in your own way. If change feels scary, good ... it's supposed to. I love this quote from Steven Pressfield: "Like self-doubt, fear is an indicator. Fear tells us what we have to do."

> You are the only person stopping you from being healthier.

The choice is yours: You can live in the safety of your labels and comfort zone, or you can expand past your current limitations.

WHAT YOU CAN DO TOMORROW

- **Filter out negative self-talk.** Your thoughts about yourself typically impact how you talk about yourself. Often, that shows up in the form of negative self-talk. One way to filter out negative self-talk is to change the person speaking and see how it makes you feel. What if the way you call yourself stupid after making a mistake were coming from your boss or advisor? How would that make you feel? Or what if the way you talk about your appearance were coming from your best friend? Would you continue to have a close relationship with that person if they persisted in demeaning you? You wouldn't put up with comments like that from your boss or friend, so you shouldn't put up with hearing your own criticisms, either. Your body is listening, even if you don't realize it. Be a good friend to yourself, especially in how you talk to yourself.

- **Improve positive self-talk.** You can combat and improve your self-talk. Be aware. What is your inner dialogue? Are you conscious of it? What beliefs do your inner voice affirm about you? Does your inner voice ever affirm who you are or what you are doing? Reflect. Picture what overcoming your mental noise will feel like. Check in with yourself and consider the thoughts you let through your filter.

- **Confront your insecurities.** Give up the illusion of control. Stop waiting on the "right" time. Do what you can with the strength you have today. Set challenging goals by visualizing a success that seems absurd right now. Focus on your strengths by leaning into what you are good at, and do it better. Invite trusted, outside perspectives to weigh in. Listen to their input without internalizing. Put structure and safeguards around your areas of weakness.

- **Ask three questions about your thoughts.** Author Jon Acuff recently wrote a book about the mental soundtracks that constantly play in the background of our minds. We might not hear them, but they are there, and they influence us in not-so-subtle ways. He talks about three questions we need to ask ourselves about our thoughts:

1. Is it true?
2. Is it helpful?
3. Is it kind?

If you answer no to any of these questions when you are stepping into an action or engaging in a thought, then it is time to reevaluate and change your decision or action. These questions have changed how I approach my thoughts and have helped me immensely as an individual, a dad, a spouse, and a business owner.

- **Ditch your labels.** It is interesting how we hate when people label us, but we love to label ourselves. We tend to find safety in the labels we pick for ourselves. But those labels often hold us back from protecting our future the way we need to. Ditch these three labels:

  1. *I'm the type of person who* _____. You are more than your horoscope or your impulses. You can change. You can adapt. You're not done growing yet.
  2. *I've always done* _____. You are more than your past. You can make new choices, take on new challenges, and create new habits.

3. *I could never do* _____. You are
   more than your fears. You can build
   courage. You can develop resilience.
   You can live fearlessly.

BUILDING MOMENTUM

After coaching more than two hundred people, I see the patterns. I see the self-doubt, the old patterns people hold on to, and the fear of letting go of aspects of their identity. I see the hesitancy to get on the scale, post progress photos, change the diet, or try a new exercise.

I also start to see an aspect of the people that they may not see within themselves. I see an ability to push through what they doubted they could do on those hard days. I see them grow into entirely new people with new habits and a new love for what their bodies can do and how to care for themselves. It's a beautiful process to witness. Here is the takeaway: The new you exists just beyond what you don't think you can do. But you'll never be able to see it if you can't conquer your mental noise.

STEP 1: **Imagine the man in the park.**

You can't stop negative thoughts from popping up, but you can choose not to listen to them. Imagine you are walking in a park just as the sun is going down. Few people are around, so you are startled when you hear a voice shouting in your direction. You look over and see a man gesturing and yelling at you wildly. As you get a bit closer, you realize he is both insulting you and demanding that you come closer. What will you do? You could go closer to him, or you could turn and find a different route through the park. We both know you'd find a new route.

The hypercritical voice in your head is just like the man in the park. Yet we often choose to listen to him and put stock in what he has to say about us. The next time you hear that voice, don't cozy up to it. Hear the danger, be attentive to why that voice is shouting at you, but don't dwell on it. Remember the man in the park and actively choose a different route of thinking.

STEP 2: Ask yourself, "So what?"

Take your biggest self-doubt, your greatest worry about what people are thinking about you. Sit with it for a minute or two and ask yourself, "So what?" I'm a people-pleaser by nature. I want people to like me and think I'm great. A fear of mine is that someone will dislike me, think my work is garbage, or express dissatisfaction with my performance. When I get caught up in that abstract fear, it helps me to ask, "So what?" So what if they don't like me or what I do. How will that impact my life in any real way? I quickly realize it won't impact me at all. Giving power to these worries ties my self-worth to the opinions of others. By taking your worries to the limit of their logical conclusions, you can shift your perspective from abstract to concrete. Playing out the logical conclusions strips your self-doubts from having power over your choices.

STEP 3: Seek accountability.

Photos often disrupt the stories we tell. This is one reason many people don't like seeing candid photos of themselves. The photo shows a different picture than what we had imagined. Accountability acts just like those photos. Accountability is a powerful tool for revealing what is happening behind the scenes. Real reflection, real accountability, can be painful at times. If you could observe yourself for a day, would you be proud of the choices you are making? Of the thoughts you are thinking? Inviting accountability into your life will confront the stories you are telling yourself repeatedly. Accountability can come from a trusted source or from a system you build for yourself. A simple daily log, a weekly check-in, or inviting regular feedback from a mentor or coach can help you keep clear snapshots of your progress. Take the time to reflect on the direction you are headed. Accountability only works if you are actively seeking it out.

STEP 4: Combat self-limiting beliefs.

Mental noise might show up in the way you self-limit. Here are three signs you're habitually self-limiting: 1) You focus on what you can't do or can't control, 2) You use the phrase "I'm the type of person who ..." or "I'm not the type of person who ..." and 3) You assume difficulty before ever trying.

To combat the first sign, actively shift your attention to what you can do and act on what you can control. It's easier said than done, but growth will happen when you push against your limits rather than grumble about them.

Targeting the second sign will require a shift in the language you use to talk about yourself. Instead of saying, "I'm the type/not the type," you can reframe it as, "I am becoming a person who …." Ask yourself, "What would the healthier version of me do?" This simple shift can alter how you relate to a new action that feels challenging right now.

The third sign is a problem of perception. You see the outcome and assume the difficulty before ever breaking it down into small actions along the way. Back in my teaching days, I often taught students who would panic about a required research paper. But when I broke down that we would spend an entire semester building their thesis, compiling research, and working through multiple drafts, most of their tension faded. Break the outcome into its building blocks and visualize what winning the first step will look like. And if it's still hard, ask yourself if you thought such an important change would feel easy or hard. This is what hard feels like. Entrepreneur and investor Alex Hormozi said, "If you can do it when it's hard, you can keep doing it under any conditions. If you only wait to start when it's easy, you'll either never start or you'll quit the moment it gets hard again (which it always does). So you might as well start when it's hard."

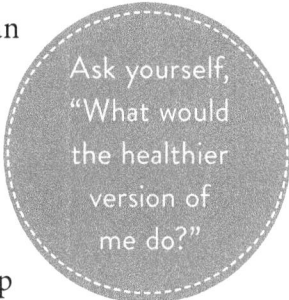

Ask yourself, "What would the healthier version of me do?"

REMOVING OBSTACLES

Here are a few common concerns for this Hack and how to address them.

I'm just hard on myself. You *think* you are hard on yourself. But ultimately, you are wired for happiness. Your mind is constantly searching for things it can use to make you feel good. If you cannot celebrate small wins (see Hack 1), you will seek alternative routes to finding happiness. For many people, this becomes destructive as they instinctively turn to substances or foods for comfort and that rush of happy hormones. For others, they turn to working overtime because they believe happiness is found in accomplishing tasks. Understand that "being hard on yourself" is a reflection of your internal desire for peace and happiness. Now, which route will truly bring more happiness: driving yourself to the edge of despair or scaling back your expectations to habits you can sustain? When you develop the habit of pushing yourself toward your goals from a place of anticipation versus a place of dread, you will thrive from the mental balance that ensues.

Negative self-talk is the only model I know. Maybe you were raised in a critical home environment. Or maybe you grew up with a parent or guardian who regularly verbalized negative thoughts about their weight, body, or appearance. It is not surprising that negative self-talk might be your default if that is the case. In addition to the strategies listed earlier, here are a few actions you can take. I call this strategy Remove/Replace/Rechoose. The first is to *remove* yourself from current negative environments as much as possible. You cannot continue feeding that monster any longer. The second option is to *replace* negative-filled spaces with ones that are made up of the type of person you aspire to be. For example, if I want to be more generous, I need to put myself in situations where there are generous people actively practicing generosity. A local charity would be the first place I would try. To be kinder to yourself and your body, look for a community of people who enjoy taking care of themselves. A local cycling club, dance studio, walking/running club, hiking group, pickleball league, or even online fitness communities are options you could test out. Try everything until you find your tribe. The third route to breaking ingrained negative self-talk is to give yourself space to *rechoose* how you talk to yourself and the language you use. Maybe you keep a thought journal. Some people find affirmations effective. I find tremendous value in faith-based teaching that speaks to my deeper identity and purpose. Remove/Replace/Rechoose will give you agency in shaping a new pattern.

I'm afraid I will fail if I start. Start anyway. Time will pass one way or another. Life is not pass/fail. Life is learning from failing. Maturing is realizing how few things truly matter and how little weight the opinions of others actually carry. Fear reveals what we value most. The best time to start is when you're afraid because then you know you have skin in the game. The downside to starting a new path is winding up right back where you started. The upside to starting a new path is unlimited. Fear and failure played a role in the very first step you took as a child. And they will play a role in the next step you take for your mental and physical health.

The hurdle in front of me is just too daunting to start. The mental hurdle of a big task is a huge deterrent to starting. But without starting, there is no progress. Start with the three T's: Target, Track, and Tool.

1. What is the first *target* you can aim for within that big task?

2. What is the way you will *track* your progress? Can you build a timeline?

3. What *tool(s)* will best help you accomplish the target? If you start here, you will find a starting place as well as a path forward. Start small, win small!

THE HACK IN ACTION

I was the kid who would practice before practice. I would visualize taking it to the rim on the basketball court or hitting a perfect cross on the soccer field for days leading up to a game. My internal drive to perform at a high level, and my ability to visualize how I'd act in certain scenarios, helped me play at my best.

But there was a flipside. The impulse to practice was often driven by the fear of looking unprepared, of feeling like a failure. The ability to visualize winning also meant I had the ability to visualize failing. Feeling like a failure, feeling worthless, or feeling like I let people down became my greatest fear. My self-worth became tied to my performance and how I thought others saw me.

My concern for appearances carried over into academics and my early career. It seemed to pay off. I played collegiate soccer, was a youth pastor, graduated with honors, was put into leadership positions as a young teacher, and won grants for my research and awards for my thesis while earning my master's degree. I wanted to be impressive, but that came at a cost.

Any hint of coming up short of my high expectations would tear me up with stress and push me into unsustainable work patterns. I would go through long stretches of neglecting sleep, proper hydration, and exercise. When I did work out, I would only do exercises that focused on moves I was already good at because I was so concerned about looking silly on an unfamiliar machine or looking weak on a new exercise. It was only after a serious low-back injury that I realized that my desire to achieve and my fears of looking like a failure were preventing me from protecting my long-term health.

I started lifting weights for the first time. Eventually, I learned more about nutrition, how to eat for my goals, and how to put boundaries around my sleep habits. I had to get out of my own way. I had to change my internal dialogue so I could stop equating failing with being a failure. Sure, I continued to prepare. I watched videos on form and nutrition, I researched and studied different workout programs, and I had to make myself complete exercises that revealed my weaknesses.

The process of training was pivotal for me to break through my fear of failure. Every day in the gym, I failed at something, and I learned that failure was a good thing. The more I saw growth through failure, the more willing I became to take risks and not internalize critique. I don't think I ever would have had the courage to risk my family's livelihood and start my own business without that growth.

|—|

Mastering the mental noise is about more than saying morning affirmations. It is about overcoming an internal resistance that wants to rob you of joy and feeling in alignment with your thoughts and actions. Spend time working on your thoughts, and you will cultivate resilience, determination, and self-belief. You will become more open to new opportunities and possibilities. Overcome self-doubt by doing the hard things even when they feel hard. This will be your new foundation for personal and professional growth, allowing you to pursue your dreams with a confidence you've built up through consistency and perseverance.

How you talk to yourself will not get easier after you continue striving for the approval of others. It will not get easier after you continue expecting perfection from yourself and others. It will not get easier after you continue drawing from dry wells. How you talk to yourself will not get easier after you continue saying *I'll do it later.* It will not get easier when you continue focusing on the things you can't control instead of the things you can. It will not get easier after you continue neglecting the basics. And how you talk to yourself will not get easier after you continue saying you'll change one of these days. Changing how you think and talk to yourself will never get easier than it is *right now*. Start today.

GIVE YOURSELF A BEDTIME

Create Better Sleep Habits to Reduce Stress

*The best bridge between despair
and hope is a good night's sleep.*
— E. JOSEPH COSSMAN, INVENTOR AND ENTREPRENEUR

THE PROBLEM: SLEEP IS AN AFTERTHOUGHT

WHAT IS YOUR first thought the moment your alarm goes off? If you are like me, you wish you could hit an indefinite snooze button and sleep until you naturally wake up. Your brain recognizes that you need more sleep and recovery before starting your day. But let's wind back the clock for a moment. What were your thoughts the two to three hours before going to sleep? You may have felt scattered, distracted, and busy completing the final tasks for the day or worrying about the tasks for the next day. At what point do you listen and respond to your brain's morning message that you need more sleep and recovery time?

Sleep is often an afterthought. In general, we do a poor job with sleep planning and setting ourselves up for proper sleep habits. We wake up with a huge desire to sleep more but then do not use our time, thoughts, or energy to ensure that we sleep better the next night. Or the next. Or the next. Sleep is relegated to a lower tier of priority than all the tasks we need to accomplish, yet it is sleep that allows us to complete those tasks. Going to sleep is our last action of the day, and we often think of it as last in importance too.

Poor sleep habits and poor sleep planning can dramatically lower one's quality of life. Depleted energy levels and reduced motivation are only scratching the surface of the detrimental impacts of under-sleeping. From a cognitive and mental health perspective, even one night of insufficient sleep noticeably impacts attention span, alertness, reaction times, information retention, and stress management. The physical side effects from a night of poor sleep move beyond low energy to reduced hormone production, higher inflammation, and weakened immune functions.

Chronic sleep deprivation has far greater consequences. Matthew Walker, author of *Why We Sleep*, put it this way: "The shorter your sleep, the shorter your life. The leading causes of disease and death in developed nations—diseases that are crippling healthcare systems, such as heart disease, obesity, dementia, diabetes, and cancer—all have recognized causal links to a lack of sleep." Chronic sleep deprivation can impair concentration, risk assessments, problem-solving skills, and overall cognitive performance. It may also increase the risk of age-related cognitive decline and neurodegenerative diseases.

Sleep struggles and poor sleep habits do not appear to be slowing down anytime soon. The global sleep aid market in 2021 was reported to be around $74 billion. Projections from Precedence Research show that number growing to $124 billion by 2030. Increasingly demanding work schedules and busy lifestyles have led to people sacrificing sleep to meet these demands. Plus, technology advancements in personal devices have led to higher levels of nighttime distractions, and increased exposure to artificial lighting and blue light has disrupted natural circadian rhythms. Greater financial stress, ever-increasing healthcare costs, and societal mental health challenges have led to a drop in average nightly sleep. You cannot afford to let poor sleep and harmful sleep habits be an afterthought any longer.

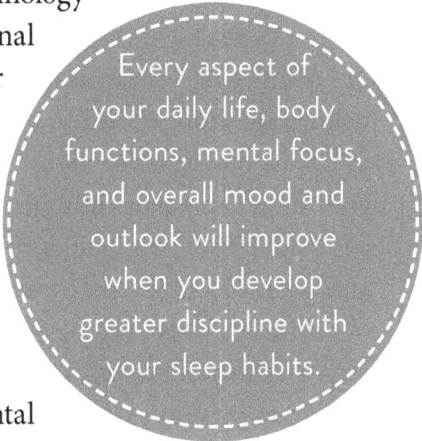

> Every aspect of your daily life, body functions, mental focus, and overall mood and outlook will improve when you develop greater discipline with your sleep habits.

THE HACK: GIVE YOURSELF A BEDTIME

My wife and I have four sons. As you can guess, we have had plenty of sleepless nights with each of them. Each son, at some point in their childhood, has pushed back on needing a bedtime. As their parents, we continue to enforce bedtime despite their often vigorous protests. We do it for them and for us. We can see the visible difference that a lack of sleep makes in their emotions, choices, mood, energy, and overall health. As adults, we can usually mask the symptoms of poor sleep better than children can, but a lack of sleep impacts us to the same degree as it impacts children.

Most of us do not have the luxury of sleeping until we wake up naturally. But we do have the knowledge of when the alarm will go off. It doesn't take a mathematician to count back seven or eight hours from the time of that alarm and set a bedtime for ourselves. So why don't we do it? You probably remember lying in bed at night, hearing the sounds of your parents, guardians, or older siblings still awake. You wished you were "big enough" to stay up as late as you wanted. As a college student or young adult, your wish came true. It is fair to say that most of us did not enter adulthood with superior sleep patterns. Recreating or adapting our sleep routines is essential at different stages of our adult lives. The best place to start, no matter what stage of life you are in, is a firm bedtime.

A firm bedtime sets a clear intention for your brain to act on. It promotes better sleep quality by ensuring an adequate duration of sleep. It improves your chances of experiencing uninterrupted deep sleep cycles, particularly the late, high REM-rich sleep (typically between the sixth and eighth hours of sleep). Having a set bedtime helps you foster a consistent sleep schedule, allowing your body the opportunity to develop a more natural sleep-wake rhythm. And finally, setting a bedtime makes you prioritize the steps needed to get to bed on time. You will naturally filter out habits that hinder getting to bed on time once you commit to protecting your sleep pattern.

It is worth your effort and time to improve your sleep quality. Sleep plays an essential role in maintaining our physical well-being. It strengthens our immune system, regulates hormones, and supports a healthy metabolism. Sufficient sleep is associated with a lower risk of developing chronic conditions like heart disease, diabetes, and obesity. It also helps regulate emotions, reduces the risk of developing mood disorders like depression and anxiety, and enhances mental well-being.

Sleep boosts our learning and memory capabilities, creativity, and problem-solving skills. During sleep, the brain consolidates information and forms new connections. It improves attention, concentration, and focus. Sleep benefits athletes and others who rely on fine motor skills and coordination, and it is vital for muscle building and fat loss. Every aspect of your daily life, body functions, mental focus, and overall mood and outlook will improve when you develop greater discipline with your sleep habits.

WHAT YOU CAN DO TOMORROW

- **Start a bedtime routine.** A consistent bedtime routine signals to the body that it's time to wind down, helping to relax the mind and prepare for sleep. Your routine does not have to be long or elaborate. Keep it simple and short to start, and then expand as you want. Here is a sample routine: Stretch, read, or pray for a few minutes. Do a quick brain dump of anything still bouncing around in your mind. Get dressed for bed. Brush your teeth. Keeping your routine the same night after night will help your brain connect those activities with the act of going to sleep.

- **Create a nighttime checklist.** Ever been at the point of falling asleep, and then you remember that you left one light on or a door unlocked? Make yourself a reusable nighttime checklist that you keep beside your bed. Physically check everything off the list each night to make sure everything is done and reassure your brain that nothing is left hanging to worry about. You can also add any items you need to have ready first thing in the morning (such as your running attire and gear) so your morning routine will go more smoothly, too.

- **Save the bed for sleeping.** Our mind connects locations to activities. Your brain will program itself to think the bed is for bingeing Netflix or snacking if that is what you do in your bed on a regular basis. It will be challenging to go to sleep if your brain expects dopamine hits and entertainment when you are in bed, trying to go to sleep. Retrain your brain by only getting in bed when you are sleepy and ready to sleep. You will benefit from falling asleep quicker and staying asleep longer.

- **Do a digital detox.** Consistent screen use and the mental stimulation from devices at night can be a major sleep disrupter. Turn off electronic devices, including smart- phones, tablets, and TVs, at least thirty minutes before bedtime to minimize your exposure to blue light and to promote relax- ation. This will give you time to transition your mind away from the digital world and implement your new bedtime routine.

BUILDING MOMENTUM

The act of consistently prioritizing sleep creates a positive feedback loop, generating momentum that reinforces your other healthy habits and further enhances sleep quality. The best fat burner is sleep. The best stress relief is sleep. The best immune booster is sleep. The best cognitive sup- port is also sleep. Once you have your bedtime set and a solid bedtime routine, there are several other pieces to address to maximize the effectiveness of your sleeping time and those amazing benefits. You can unlock the transformative power of consistent deep sleep and make every other area of your health journey easier and more sustainable than ever.

STEP 1: Optimize your sleep environment.

Your sleep environment plays a major role in the quality and length of your sleep. Make sure your bedroom is cool, dark, and quiet. Adjust the temperature to bring your body temperature down. One of the main reasons we wake up during the night is because our body temperature increases. Keeping your room cool, with blankets that you can remove if you get warm, is the best way to maintain a cool body temperature throughout the night.

Keeping the room dark will help you sleep deeper. Think about using blackout curtains or an eye mask, particularly in seasons of the year with the highest average daylight. To maintain a quiet sleeping environment, consider using earplugs or a white noise machine to create a peaceful space and minimize noise disruptions.

Avoid bright overhead lights after 10 p.m. Minimize screen time and blue light as much as possible after dark. Sleep experts recommend time in the morning and evening in natural sunlight when possible. Experiment with essential oils known for their relaxing properties, such as lavender and chamomile. Use a diffuser or apply a few drops on a fabric or pillowcase to create a soothing scent in your sleep environment.

STEP 2: Add micronutrients.

Micronutrient supplementation can be an effective method for most people to improve the quality of their sleep. You might do better without supplements, with one, or with a sleep blend. It's worth your time to figure out what is best for you. I recommend starting with your bedtime and sleep environment and then adding one supplement at a time as you see fit and with consultation from a trusted physician or nutrition coach.

Magnesium is a required mineral responsible for over three hundred chemical reactions within the body, some of which impact sleep and muscle relaxation. A lot of data suggests magnesium can aid with relaxation and sleep quality. Daily supplementation has been shown to improve natural melatonin production and increase sleep time. Experts recommend magnesium threonate or magnesium bisglycinate to best aid sleep. Try taking around 200 milligrams one hour before bed.

The best stress relief is sleep. The best immune booster is sleep. The best cognitive support is also sleep.

L-theanine is an incredible amino acid supplement found naturally in green tea. Its primary use in the evening is to enhance relaxation and sleep and reduce cortisol and stress levels. Try taking around 200 milligrams one hour before bed.

Apigenin is one of the most widely researched flavonoids, and it functions as an antioxidant and has anti-inflammatory effects. It is found in many vegetables, herbs, and fruits and is useful for sleep as a natural relaxant and stress reliever. Try taking around 50 milligrams one hour before bed.

I typically avoid melatonin supplementation. Most people produce adequate levels of melatonin naturally, and melatonin supplements are a poorly regulated market. Short-term use can be effective for shift workers or jet lag, but long-term supplementation is unnecessary unless medically prescribed. For all supplementation, seek the input of a trusted medical expert.

STEP 3: Set boundaries on alcohol and caffeine.

Caffeine is an effective and well-researched stimulant. I am not trying to take away your coffee. In fact, coffee is a fantastic delivery system for caffeine. The dose and the timing of your caffeine intake are what really matters. In simple terms, caffeine is a blocking agent that tricks your brain into thinking it's not tired. Researchers have shown that caffeine has a half-life of six hours. This means that six hours after caffeine consumption, half of that caffeine is still active in your system. Even if you are able to fall asleep, the blocking ability of caffeine is still active and can inhibit deep recovery sleep. Try to eliminate caffeine intake eight to ten hours before your bedtime to ensure the lasting impact of caffeine has worn off. As for a recommended total caffeine intake, note that each person will have a different reaction. Some people have high noticeable sensitivity, and others have a low noticeable sensitivity. In general, a caffeine intake of 400 milligrams (roughly four cups of coffee) or less per day is a solid recommendation.

Alcohol, on the other hand, is classified as a sedative, and many people attempt to use it as a relaxant or even as a sleep aid. But alcohol is a major sleep disrupter, even if it can seem to help some people fall asleep. True restorative sleep and the sedation brought on by outside sources are two entirely different mechanisms in the brain. Alcohol will disrupt and greatly diminish the quality of your sleep compared to natural sleep, even causing you to fully wake up multiple times per night.

Alcohol consumption reduces growth hormone release, which mostly happens when we sleep and is vital for tissue building and tissue repair. Alcohol is effectively a poison that creates stress on our system, leads to cellular damage, and impacts inflammation levels. Regular consumption destroys your natural gut microbiome and severely disrupts a healthy hormonal balance as a result. As a fitness professional, I regularly advise my clients to remove alcoholic beverages from their lives as much as possible. If you choose to make alcohol consumption a part of your life, do so mindfully. Placing a boundary of one to two drinks per week might seem restrictive, but if your goal is sustainable health, along with better sleep, it is a wise course of action.

REMOVING OBSTACLES

Here are a few common concerns for this Hack and how to address them.

I set a bedtime, but I can't fall asleep. Give it time. Your body and mind will need several weeks to adjust to a new pattern and bedtime. Think of lying in bed at a consistent time, whether you "feel" sleepy or not, as training yourself to sleep. Over time, you will notice that the duration of time from when your head hits the pillow to when you drift off into deep sleep will shorten. Use that time for prayer, reflection, or deep breathing.

I can't turn my brain off at night. Complete your nighttime checklist. Read something that relaxes you and takes you out of your normal decision-making mindset. Do a brain dump where you write out every thought you have over a three-to-five-minute period. Make time for yoga or stretching, and add prayer or meditation to your nighttime routine to help relax your mind. Dive into aromatherapy options to reduce stress in the evening. You can find many apps and tranquility channels on YouTube that can help quiet your mind. Test out what works for you and be ready to adapt as needed.

I don't want to put rules around my sleep. You already have rules about how you sleep, but they may not be effective or beneficial ones. I remember being thirty years old, a teacher, and waiting tables nights and weekends to make ends meet for my growing family. I was overworked and stressed, but I looked and felt younger than the servers in their early twenties because I slept six to seven hours a night and drank mostly water. They stayed up drinking after their shifts, and they barely slept. They used energy drinks to keep going. You are probably saying, "I'm not as bad as that." Well, that's good—then you have some boundaries already. What this Hack is all about is making those boundaries a little bit better. Don't think you have to do everything all at once. Find one simple swap, one simple thing you can do better to sleep better. You can build and add from there.

I have small children. So, what about me? This is a challenge. Here are a few actions you can take. 1) Lower your expectations: your body can adapt to less sleep for a season.

2) Sync your sleep schedule: maybe you'll have an earlier bedtime for a time. 3) Take turns: if you have a partner, plan to swap roles if possible. 4) Naps are your friend: naps, whenever possible, can be incredible to help you get by when sleep is disrupted. 5) Put extra time into reducing stress: see Hack 7 for details on how to handle your stress.

THE HACK IN ACTION

As a twenty-five-year-old graduate student, Sarah was willing to do whatever she had to do to keep up with both her demanding course load and her part-time job. As she juggled classes, research projects, twenty hours a week of off-campus work, and various personal commitments, sleep had become a luxury she felt she couldn't afford. Determined to excel in her studies and career, she convinced herself that sacrificing sleep and relying on large amounts of caffeine was a necessary trade-off for a time.

Halfway into her first year of grad school, Sarah was averaging four to five hours of sleep per night, with the occasional all-nighter the day before a large research paper was due. She brushed off the fatigue she was experiencing and relied on coffee and energy drinks to get her through the day. She believed that as long as she pushed through her exhaustion, she could manage the workload and meet her deadlines. After all, many of her classmates and colleagues seemed to be doing the same, normalizing the notion that less sleep equaled more productivity.

However, as time went on, Sarah began to notice some serious impacts of her lack of sleep. She found herself grappling with persistent gut health issues, experiencing frequent bouts of indigestion and bloating. The combination of sleep deprivation and excessive caffeine intake had taken a toll on her digestive system, and she couldn't ignore the impact it was having on her overall health.

Moreover, Sarah started noticing other signs of distress in her body. Stress responses became more pronounced. She developed several eye infections and was sick far more often. Mental fog seemed to settle in every day, impairing her ability to concentrate and perform at her best. Anxiety levels soared, making Sarah feel more and more out of sorts and unable to relax even after passing major deadlines.

As she reflected on these changes, Sarah realized the cost of neglecting her sleep was far higher than she had ever imagined. The realization hit her hard—her physical health, mental well-being, and academic performance were all compromised by her misguided belief that quality sleep was optional.

With a newfound determination to prioritize her well-being, Sarah resolved to make a change. She committed to establishing a consistent sleep schedule, setting aside dedicated time for rest and rejuvenation. She reduced her reliance on caffeine and sought healthier alternatives to manage her energy levels throughout the day.

After several weeks, Sarah's gut health improved, stress responses subsided, mental clarity returned, and anxiety levels began to ease. She understood that a well-rested mind and body were not luxuries but prerequisites for achieving success and maintaining long-term well-being.

Sarah's story serves as a powerful reminder that sacrificing sleep for the sake of productivity is a flawed approach. By valuing her sleep and taking care of herself, she discovered a renewed sense of vitality, balance, and resilience—a testament to the transformative power of prioritizing rest.

⊩⊢⊣⊪

Sleep can either be your superpower or your weak link. The simplest way to improve your life expectancy and quality of life is to improve your sleep. The "I'll sleep when I'm dead" way of thinking is no longer viable. We have myriad data and studies that show the absolute havoc wrecked by chronic sleep deprivation. Anecdotally, I have experienced changes in my stress levels, mental health, and gut health in seasons where sleep was limited (after the birth of a child, for example) compared to seasons where quality sleep was abundant. Even if you only increase your sleep by five minutes a night, after twelve days, you will be sleeping an hour more than before. Small changes can lead to major benefits quickly. Small wins lead to big health.

Quality sleep cannot be an afterthought any longer. I was a high school teacher for many years, and I saw the mental health of my students dip year after year. Informal polling showed startling results about their sleep habits. I remember one year, I polled forty high school seniors, and only nine out of forty said they slept more than five hours per night. Most of them looked at me like I was crazy when I talked about their need for eight to ten hours as young adults. When more adults understand the importance of deep sleep and model that behavior for their loved ones, kids, friends, and peers, then our society will become healthier and more hopeful. Start with you, but don't stop with you.

MOVE WELL FOR MORE LIFE

Protect Your Mobility and Strength to Unlock the World

If you are in a bad mood, go for a walk.
If you are still in a bad mood, go for another walk.
— HIPPOCRATES, PHILOSOPHER

THE PROBLEM: EXERCISE IS SEEN AS PUNISHMENT

YOU MAY HAVE said or heard one of these statements:
"I need to work out to burn off all that food I just ate."

"I'm going for a run later to earn that cookie."

"No pain, no gain."

"That workout made me so sore, so it must have been a really good workout."

Each of these comments frames exercise as a form of punishment for choices or implies that exercise has to feel miserable or painful to "count."

The exercise-as-punishment model is a pervasive norm in today's society. Youth sports teams often get assigned extra sprints or exercises as a consequence of poor performance. Adults often think they need to do extra exercises because they enjoyed a dessert or treat, and they feel guilty if they don't "burn those calories off." This mindset creates a barrier to leading a healthy and active lifestyle. When exercise is associated with negative feelings such as guilt and obligation, or as a means to counteract indulgences, it becomes challenging to develop a consistent and sustainable fitness routine.

One key problem is that perceiving exercise as punishment sets up a negative cycle of self-punishment and negative reinforcement. You might try to engage in intense or grueling workouts to make up for indulgent behavior or to meet unrealistic body image standards. This punitive approach often leads to feelings of inadequacy and burnout, creating a negative relationship with exercise.

Furthermore, when exercise is viewed as punishment, it becomes a chore rather than a choice. You begin to feel forced into engaging in physically demanding activity, resulting in a lack of motivation and enjoyment. When movement becomes associated with drudgery, your motivation and willpower will suffer tremendously. For many, this can lead to a sedentary lifestyle, contributing to various health issues such as osteoporosis, heart disease, and mental health disorders.

Physical activity has numerous mental health benefits, including reducing stress, anxiety, and depression. However, if exercise is seen as a burden, the potential positive effects on mental health are diminished. Thoughts of self-loathing, shame, or guilt during exercise strip away many of the positive mental impacts exercise provides.

The exercise-as-punishment model also makes many people believe that their movement needs to live up to the high expectations of the fitness industry that they see in gyms, in group classes, or on social media. This misconception feeds the myth that exercise must feel rigorous, be painful, or cause high levels of soreness for it to "count." It also creates a high barrier of entry to people who never felt good at sports or athletics when they were young or who haven't been active for quite some time. Instead of a choice, exercise feels like a chore. Instead of a source of joy, exercise feels like an ordeal to endure. Instead of a sign of freedom, exercise becomes a symbol of mental entrapment.

THE HACK: MOVE WELL FOR MORE LIFE

It's time to reframe exercise away from the punishment model. Exercise is movement with purpose. There is no "right" way to move your body, and there is no predetermined purpose for that movement. You have thousands of options to choose from with an infinite range of purposes. The goal is to depressurize how we think about exercise. The more we begin to see movement as a source of joy rather than a cost we pay, the more we will choose to move and enjoy our lives.

Movement is a source of freedom. Even those most averse to the idea of exercise do not want to lose the possibility of movement. Movement is one of the first abilities we take for granted and one of the most painful and missed abilities once it is lost. A preventable back injury when I was twenty-eight was my wake-up call to how much I needed to protect my body and mobility. At the time, I was a teacher, soccer coach, and dad of three young boys. I spent close to a week unable to get out of bed and three weeks in pain and unable to play with my kids. Nothing is as gut-wrenching as trying to explain to a four-year-old why Daddy can't wrestle with him or pick him up. That was the moment I committed to doing everything in my power to get stronger and take my health seriously. Having more mobility and strength is about having more freedom. And specifically, the freedom to take part in a wider range of opportunities that bring enjoyment and connection.

> Being more fit is about having more capacity to enjoy life.

Being more fit, having more mobility, and being stronger are not about *looking* more fit. Fitness, in and of itself, is not the end goal. Being more fit is about having more capacity to enjoy life. Social media might make it seem that health is all about appearances, but it goes much deeper than that. When we reframe movement as enjoyment, we realize that every form of activity is a statement celebrating what our bodies can do while also protecting our ability to prolong doing what brings us joy. Playing sports with my boys, modeling an active lifestyle for them, and helping many other people develop a greater love for movement and exercise bring me incredible joy. Workouts that once felt like a task to accomplish now feel like a path to a more fulfilling life!

Exercise can and should be fun. What movement makes your body and mind feel good? Do you enjoy it? If you can answer those two questions, you have an activity that you can use to build your foundation of regular, healthy movement. When we find activities that align with our interests, such as dancing, hiking, or team sports, then exercise becomes a source of pleasure. Engaging in activities we genuinely enjoy not only makes us more likely to participate but also provides a sense of fulfillment and accomplishment, boosting our overall well-being. The truly amazing side effect is that you will begin to discover that other activities that once felt daunting now seem doable and worth exploring. This is what I mean when I say that exercise unlocks doors that you never even noticed before.

Perceiving exercise as enjoyable nurtures a positive relationship with our bodies. Instead of focusing on weight loss or conforming to societal standards, we can appreciate our bodies for their strength, resilience, and capacity to move. This shift in perspective fosters a sense of gratitude and a healthier body image, leading to improved mental and emotional well-being. Of course, increased exercise will play a role in weight management and cardiovascular health. And weight training will benefit muscle building, joint and bone health, and strength. All of those results are much easier to attain when seen as a byproduct of a healthy lifestyle versus the sole objective of exercise.

Finally, embracing exercise as a source of enjoyment promotes a holistic approach to wellness. Physical activity releases endorphins, neurotransmitters that induce feelings of pleasure and reduce stress. By incorporating exercise into our daily lives in a way that brings us joy, we can reduce anxiety, boost our moods, and enhance our cognitive abilities. The positive effects extend beyond the gym or class, allowing us to tackle daily challenges with a greater sense of resilience and clarity. The mobility, strength, and mental focus you build during exercise transfers to all other aspects of your life, bringing your mindful approach to self-care to the forefront in every situation you face.

WHAT YOU CAN DO TOMORROW

- **Go for five minutes.** Maybe you are an overthinker like me. Maybe you spend a lot of time in indecision, trying to find *the* best thing and not just acting on *one* of many right things. Just get moving. Action always supersedes fear and indecision. Set a timer for five minutes and just start. Your brain will catch up to your body once your body is in motion. When the five minutes are up, check in with yourself. Do you feel like you can go on? I promise that 99 percent of the time, you will answer yes. And if you need to answer no, then be proud of doing five minutes. Five minutes is always more than zero minutes. It's a win-win either way.

- **Start with fun.** Maybe starting is the hardest part for you. Reduce the friction around exercise by starting with a movement you truly enjoy. You will quickly notice your stress, anxiousness, and mental fog decrease as your mood and energy levels rise. Enjoy walking? Find a great walking location or setup. Love dancing? Pick an energizing song and get after it. Does stretching relax your mind? Download a yoga app or find stretching videos online and turn your living room into an instant relaxation zone. Focus on building your foundation and celebrate your small victories.

- **Mix it up.** Maybe you're afraid of falling into old, destructive exercise habits. You do not have to exercise the way you used to. It might be time to try a new activity. You could try a sport you've always thought looked fun. You could try a movement that's silly and outside your comfort zone. You could try an activity that you enjoyed as a kid (roller skating, anyone?). Maybe you could finally try out that hobby someone in your friend group is always talking about.

- **Create a challenge.** Need to get the competitive juices flowing? I like to encourage my clients to set up small challenges for themselves. Here are a few examples that might work for you: 1) Step challenge: try to hit or exceed that number of steps. 2) Timed challenge: try to do a particular exercise for a specific amount of time. An example is to hold a plank for sixty seconds. 3) Speed challenge: try to complete a task under a certain time limit. 4) Weight challenge: try to lift a new higher weight range on an exercise you have experience doing. 5) Balance challenge: test your balance by brushing your teeth while standing on one leg (switch legs halfway through), by a standing exercise (a single-leg deadlift, for example), by a floor exercise (the bird dog pose is great), or by sitting on a stability ball while working. 6) Jump challenge: pick up that dust-covered jump rope and set a rep target. Or you could practice skipping, box jumps, or single-leg hops. The opportunities are endless. Start with an activity you can do safely, and make it more rewarding with a target.

BUILDING MOMENTUM

The key to long-term strength and mobility is progression. Weightlifters spend a lot of time talking about progressive overload. In basic terms, progressive overload means increasing at least one variable of the exercise to make it more challenging over time. I like to apply this to all forms of movement as the concept of "repetition without repetition." Your body is adaptive to the signals you send, but it will stop adapting if you only send the same signals over and over. This section is all about increasing the strength of the signals you send your body over time so you never feel stuck or miss out on unlocking that next opportunity.

STEP 1: Set big fitness goals that have nothing to do with the scale.

There is nothing wrong with weight loss (or weight gain) goals for some people. But I find that for many people, having only weight goals and using exercise as a tool to achieve them leads to unnecessary pressure and frustration. Weight change can be on the periphery of your efforts, but setting fitness goals that you have full control over is a far more balanced approach and allows you to see the broad benefits of increased fitness instead of just one measurement.

One of my clients knew he needed to lose weight. He had tried and struggled several times. During one of our early conversations, he told me he had always wanted to say he could run a mile without stopping. We decided to make that our primary goal and not weight loss. He knew losing weight would help, but he wasn't fixated on the scale or beating himself up if his weight didn't go down. We began building up his strength and muscular endurance, increasing his daily steps and adding in more walking over time. When he felt confident, he started adding jogging into his walks. One of my best days as a coach was when he messaged me to say that he had jogged a full mile without walking! He had also lost about twenty pounds on the path to that one mile. But which achievement do you think made him most proud? Yep, running the mile mattered far more. For now and forever, he will know he's the guy who ran a mile when he never thought he could. That says far more about him than a number on a scale ever will.

STEP 2: Have a plan ... with a backup plan.

You are a creature of habit. Without a plan of how to progress, you will quickly do the same thing repeatedly, day after day. That can work just fine for sustaining but will not be effective for progressing. You will not see growth in your strength and mobility without signaling to your body that growth is needed. That will require gradually changing the stimuli, or "repetition without repetition," so your body can keep pace while also adapting. The easiest way to ensure progress without feeling overwhelmed is to have an actual plan for progression.

Most gym-goers inherently know the value of a progressive plan because they are trained to walk into the gym with a training plan. They follow the plan and track their progress. They increase their sets, repetitions, and weight selection, and they improve their form. This is a highly effective strategy to build growth in the gym. If you are a gym-goer and have never used a training plan, I highly recommend you take the time to build a plan. Find a quality plan that is appropriate for your level or, even better, hire a professional to build a personalized plan for you. You can apply a progressive plan to other types and forms of movements as well.

Let's break down a simple approach:

- Start with your **big fitness goals** (yes, the ones that have nothing to do with the scale). What skills do you need to achieve each goal? Write them down.

- Now, what **consistent behaviors/habits** do you need to nail down to build each of those skills? Write them down.

- Last, what **small, daily actions** do you need to perform to master those behaviors? Write them down.

Your actions are now your daily action plan. Over time, your actions will build your habits, your habits will build your skills, and your skills will help you accomplish your goals. Focusing on the goal leads to frustration and anxiety. Focusing on the actions leads to controlling the controllables.

But you still need a backup plan. Mike Tyson said it best: "Everyone has a plan till they get punched in the mouth." What is your backup for when life surprises you? Imagine being a quarterback in a football game and calling a passing play. You will know the primary route you want to throw. You'd love a touchdown with every pass. But you'd be a fool to think the defense would give you that gift each time. A good quarterback knows his checkdowns. When option one is covered, he moves to option two, then three. And sometimes, he just has to get rid of the ball and call another play altogether. He would rather get a few yards than zero yards, and he would rather get zero than go negative yards. Have your checkdowns. They can be easy considerations, such as: "If I can't get to the gym, I will stretch at home" or "If the pickleball league gets rained out, I will go for a twenty-minute walk." You can always find options that give you a win, even if it's not the win you originally planned.

STEP 3: Measure and adapt.

Nothing great was ever built by default. Some results in history have been accidental (penicillin is a great example), but the effort to attempt and adapt was intentional. You will not wake up one day and be healthy by accident. Neglect always leads to dysfunction and never leads to improvement. To make sure your actions are building you closer to your goals, you need to have clear ways to measure growth and progress. The way you measure depends on your goals. If your goal is to be an Olympic skier, you will need fairly exhaustive measurements. But if your goal is sustainable health, you can be more relaxed. *Do I feel better? Do I look better? Do I have more energy? Do I have an improved mood? Am I less stressed? Am I happier? Am I stronger? Do I feel proud of my efforts?* Those are a few sample questions that can help you measure your progress.

What if you are putting more energy into movement but not seeing positive results, or those results are fading? That is a signal that it is time to adapt. Sometimes, what we think we need to do isn't actually what we need to do. And that's okay. The sooner we recognize the disconnect between our actions and goals, the sooner we can attempt a new route. The simplest way to adapt is to create consistent feedback loops. A tree has incredible feedback loops that constantly signal messages from the environment so that the tree makes small adjustments to grow in better directions to get more sunlight. Feedback loops are vital to coaching relationships and mentorships. You will see more growth when you get better feedback more often and more consistently. Find or build your feedback loops.

REMOVING OBSTACLES

Here are a few common concerns for this Hack and how to address them.

I'm nervous about going to the gym. That used to be me, too. Here are the tips that helped me overcome fear at the gym. First: Prepare. Write out your main objective for the workout and where you will start your first exercise. Maybe you want to get your heart rate to a certain zone. Maybe you hit two chest exercises. Or maybe you want to focus on improving your mobility. Have a ten-minute plan focused on the objective. Once that is done, the pressure is off because you hit your objective already.

Second: Practice. For your first workout, don't even try

to work out. Your goal is to walk through the gym and acclimate (I still do this at a new gym). Try out a machine or two, hit a stationary bike or treadmill, and call it a day. For your first month, center your workouts around moves you feel most comfortable with. A month in, and you will feel much more confident to try new moves. Watch demos of new exercises at home and visualize yourself doing the movements.

Third: Shift your perspective. Remind yourself that this is about you, not anyone else. Remember, no one is watching you because everyone is just as preoccupied with their own internal dialogue and appearance as you are. Imagine you're just doing another activity that you enjoy and you don't feel pressure to perform.

I'm concerned about former injuries or getting injured. Safety is the most important consideration with any exercise plan. But here is the harsh reality: not exercising is far more dangerous for your health than exercising. An abundance of studies show that all-cause mortality rates are dramatically higher for sedentary populations than for active ones. Often, people will express concern about strength training as an injury risk. Let's look at just one way (there are many) that resistance training reduces injury risk factors: your bones. When you lift weights, you signal to your body that it needs to reinforce your bones to withstand outside forces. A balanced diet combined with resistance training is the best prevention tactic for osteoporosis. The risk of occasionally pulling a muscle is far less than the risk of living for years with brittle bones. And as mentioned previously, you can find an almost unlimited variety of safe exercise formats. Speak to an exercise specialist if you have concerns, but do not let fear prevent you from living your best life.

I feel like I'm a hopeless cause when it comes to exercise. That is a value statement. A value statement is something you believe that guides your thoughts and actions. You can believe a value statement with some evidence, poor evidence, or even no evidence, but your belief does not make it true. Something in your background has led you to believe that you are not "good" at exercise or that exercise isn't fun. But that doesn't make you hopeless. I am guessing you would never say you're a hopeless cause when it comes to being a little kinder to people. I bet you believe you could be a little kinder to people if you practiced it and focused on it. The same is true for exercise. What you give your attention to grows. If you give your attention to limiting beliefs about your abilities, those limiting beliefs will grow. When you give your attention to moving the best you can now and focusing on expanding your ability, it will grow! You can move a little more and a little better tomorrow than you did today.

THE HACK IN ACTION

Stephen let a tragic accident and major spinal surgery keep him away from exercise for too long. And I can't blame him. He was a well-respected firefighter. He was training new hires on the station's bucket truck when the hydraulic boom failed and the bucket truck he was in fell over fifty feet onto pavement. Stephen, his family, friends, and medical team believe it is a miracle of God that he survived that fall. Even more amazing is that he regained the ability to walk after spinal fusion surgeries. He didn't take that for granted, but understandably so, he was fearful of doing anything that could cause another injury.

Stephen was wise to be cautious. Being reckless could end his life quickly, but being overly cautious could end his life slowly. His body adapted to his new normal in both positive and detrimental ways. He regained the ability to play with his small children, to hike, and to swim. But he also gained weight due to a less active lifestyle, and his bloodwork started to indicate red flags for a man in his early thirties. Five years after the injury, Stephen still did not have the confidence to get back into the exercise he had once loved.

You can move a little more and a little better tomorrow than you did today.

That's when we met, and he told me his story. He also told me that he wanted to honor God for healing his body. He wanted to be the active father his children deserved, to regain his strength, and to overcome the fear that had kept him down for far too long. And so, with unwavering determination, he committed to the process.

At the time of this writing, Stephen and I have been training together for just over a year. We started small and began gradually rebuilding his strength. We threw out the way he had trained as a high school football player and instead worked on mobility exercises, corrective exercises, and strength training tailored to his condition. Three days a week, he pushed himself a little further, conquering fears and getting the small wins bit by bit.

What Stephen has overcome is nothing short of extraordinary. He transformed his habits and his mental toughness. He is getting stronger month by month. When traveling for business, he misses the gym and now hits workouts solo whenever he can. Stephen used to wake up stressed, checking email right away and doing nothing to take care of himself before taking care of his responsibilities. He recently told me that waking up at 5:00 a.m. to work out, hit a cold shower, and have time alone with God is his idea of the best Monday morning ever.

Stephen's journey is not just about physical transformation; it is also about reclaiming his life. Anyone who has dealt with back issues can get inspired by Stephen to press on. Stephen demonstrates that even in the face of adversity, you can emerge stronger. His wife, kids, peers, and employees are witnessing the incredible power of determination, resilience, and faith he displays.

।⊢।

Simon Sinek talks about playing the infinite game. Infinite games are aspects of life that have no finish lines. Health does not have a finish line. Movement, strength, and mobility do not have finish lines. You can win or lose a game of Monopoly, but you cannot win at being a generous person. Infinite games are an ever-expanding state of being. Here's what I mean: The results in life that truly matter are not what you've done but who you are becoming. Are you in the process of becoming more mobile? Stronger? Are you learning to enjoy movement more? If yes, then you

Small Wins, Big Health

are winning at moving well for more life. But you'll never achieve total victory. There will always be more small victories, setbacks, and accomplishments ahead. That is what makes protecting your health so frustrating and rewarding at the same time. Enjoy the wins when it's easy, and celebrate your efforts when it's hard.

TAME YOUR STRESS
Find Control When Life Is Messy

I am rather like a mosquito in a nudist camp; I know what I want to do, but I don't know where to begin.
— DAVID ALLEN, AUTHOR OF *GETTING THINGS DONE*

THE PROBLEM: WE TRY TO AVOID STRESS BUT ONLY AVOID ADDRESSING OUR STRESSORS

WE KNOW STRESS is unavoidable, yet we live like we can avoid it. We create most of our targets and plans for our health in a false reality where nothing comes up, life doesn't derail us, and stress doesn't accumulate. But then the inevitable happens, and we are blindsided by external circumstances and internal pressures that we never anticipated. We fail to activate good stress to maintain consistency, and we let bad stress build to debilitating levels.

While it's natural to seek comfort and relief from stress, solely focusing on avoidance is counterproductive. Instead of creating strategies to manage our stressors, we mask them with extra layers of tasks we think will make us healthy. And all the while, those underlying stressors are getting more entrenched in our lives. It won't be long until they resurface stronger and more debilitating than ever. And they will grow at a pace beyond our ability to cover them up.

Unaddressed stressors, combined with poor coping mechanisms, are a recipe for bad stress. I define bad stress as ongoing, elevated stress levels that produce consistent negative responses. Some of these responses are voluntary, but often, they are involuntary. These responses may show up visibly, but many are only internal reactions. As a full-time graduate student and young dad, I was on the bad-stress carousel. On top of a full courseload in a thesis track program, my graduate studies funding required me to work a twenty-hour-a-week assistantship for my institute. But we needed more income to make ends meet, so I also took on another twenty hours of part-time work at a local print shop. I was stretched to the maximum with the reading, writing, and research of my courses, and I regularly slept three to five hours per night. On an external level, I appeared to be doing just fine. But internally, the accumulation of stress was wreaking havoc on my body and nervous system. I lost my appetite, and my weight continued to go down. I was plagued by constant thoughts of failure. I developed consistent gastrointestinal pain and digestive problems, and I felt unable to relax.

By the end of those two years, I knew things had to change. Although I graduated with honors, I had potential publications on the table, and my dream of pursuing a PhD in history was right in front of me, it was clear to my wife and me that our family and my physical health could not endure another four years of that pace. I had to address the stressors and learn healthier outlets for my stress.

Hard work wasn't the problem for me. The buildup of chronic stress was the problem. Chronic stress, or long-term stress, is prolonged or excessive stress that is detrimental to your health and fitness. It leads to elevated cortisol levels, which can result in weight fluctuations, muscle loss, and increased fat storage, making it more challenging to achieve fitness goals. It can hinder your body's ability to recover from workouts. Sleep disturbances and high stress levels can impede muscle repair and growth. Chronic stress is different from anxiety disorders, which require medical intervention or counseling, but the felt impact can be just as detrimental.

Telling someone dealing with bad stress to "just relax" is pointless. Their body is incapable of autoregulating stress responses and can depend on high cortisol levels to keep up with normal functions. Escapism often seems like the best path forward. Many people imagine a vacation will fix their stress, but without changing the stressors, a week off will have little to no effect on bad stress. This can lead to a perpetual cycle where temporary escapes, like binge-watching TV or overeating, become habitual and ineffective ways of coping.

Escapism merely masks the symptoms of stress rather than resolving the root causes. Furthermore, the longer stressors go unaddressed, the more they can accumulate and potentially snowball into more significant problems.

Neglected work-related stress, for example, can lead to burnout, affecting not only one's professional life but also personal well-being and relationships. Stress addicts are much more likely to develop other addictions, like substance abuse or eating disorders.

Failure to address stressors can also limit personal growth and resilience. The inability to rest and relax, along with poor sleep, means that your mental and physical growth is hampered by a reduced recovery capacity. This will impact every bodily system, including memory, focus, immunity, sex drive, metabolism, and emotional responses.

Ultimately, avoiding stress without managing its root causes is like putting a Band-Aid on a wound without treating the infection underneath. It may provide temporary relief, but it doesn't lead to healing. We must address and manage long-term stress at the source.

THE HACK: TAME YOUR STRESS

Stress is unavoidable, and it is also necessary. We cannot survive without stress, and we cannot thrive without it. Stress is not the enemy. Our response to stress via our coping mechanisms, and a gradual buildup of stress from ignoring our stressors, is what we must gain control over. The solution is to learn to be in control of our stress. The goal for sustainable health is to use good stress coupled with good stress responses. But for that, we need to dive into how stress works in our body and the effective means of handling it.

The sympathetic nervous system (SNS) is responsible for your fight-or-flight response. When you are stressed, your SNS signals your adrenal glands to release adrenaline and cortisol. This is an essential process for survival and for responding to your environment. Whether you know it or not, your SNS is always "on" to help you maintain a sense of internal balance and readiness.

Cortisol is vital to your energy and productivity. In an ideal world, your cortisol gradually rises in the early morning hours to wake you up. Within an hour of waking, your cortisol will be at its highest levels, helping you feel alert, motivated, and expectant. By midday, those levels dip to half of your peak, but you should continue to have enough energy to maintain productivity into the evening. In the late evening, your levels should be significantly lower and continue to decrease as you go from initial sleep into deep sleep.

Many of your body's systems work in opposing pairs. The bicep performs arm flexion, and the tricep performs an arm extension. Insulin, released by the pancreas, lowers blood sugar levels, but the pancreas also makes glucagon, which prevents your blood sugar from dropping too low. When the body overheats, it cools down through sweating. Conversely, when the body is too cold, it generates heat through shivering. Your parasympathetic nervous system (PNS) works in contrast to your sympathetic nervous system to "rest and digest." The PNS promotes relaxation and recovery after a stressor has passed. It facilitates activities like digestion, repair, and energy conservation.

To summarize: The sympathetic nervous system prepares the body for action and alertness, while the parasympathetic nervous system promotes rest and recovery. This balance is crucial for overall physiological and psychological well-being.

You need to know how to tap into both, and in particular, you need to develop more abilities to activate your PNS.

The first avenue you can take to activate your PNS is with your thought patterns. Think of a time when you experienced physical discomfort from a stressor in your life. Maybe it was a verbal altercation. Maybe someone cut you off in a line. How long did the discomfort last? If it was more than a few minutes, then I have news for you: it wasn't the initial event that caused the continued discomfort; it was your mind replaying it. Cortisol only has a half-life of seventy to ninety seconds in your system. Your response should have lasted a minute and a half, max. But your mind can play on an infinite loop. Every time you replay the event, your body will respond just as it did that first time. I bet you could make yourself feel physically ill right now by replaying it over again in your mind or by telling the story to someone else. Your brain doesn't know the difference.

You must stop the loop. I often remind my clients to take their thoughts captive. You do not have to be a victim to a thought pattern that creates a stress response. Taking thoughts captive means you have agency in the thoughts you allow to run free in your mind and the ones you put boundaries around. Play it out. What is the chain reaction, both mentally and physically, of negative thought patterns? How long can you continue to spiral in stress and cortisol if you allow those thoughts to go unchecked? For far, far too long. Compare that to the chain reaction you experience when you use your favorite relaxation methods to activate the parasympathetic system. Which pattern do you want to feed on purpose?

WHAT YOU CAN DO TOMORROW

- **Plan PNS activities.** Practicing parasympathetic activities offers numerous benefits when it comes to managing and reducing stress. First, PNS techniques, such as mindfulness and meditation, promote mental clarity and emotional stability, allowing individuals to respond to stressors with greater resilience. These practices encourage a state of relaxation, reducing the production of stress hormones like cortisol. One of my most recommended tools is gratitude journaling, where you dedicate a few minutes each day to write down what you're grateful for. This practice can shift your focus toward positive experiences and encourage a more optimistic outlook.

    Other excellent PNS activities you can start adding to your day include:

    deep breathing
    slow stretching
    non-competitive play
    physical intimacy
    prayer
    laughter
    green tea

massage

positive affirmations

acts of kindness

self-compassion

visualization of positive outcomes

separation of big tasks into smaller steps

encouraging voices

quality foods

sleep

exploration of ideas you are curious about

investment in social connections

Finding even five to ten minutes in your day to activate your parasympathetic system will hugely pay off in minimizing the impact of daily stress.

- **Get all types of grounding.** Grounding techniques are coping mechanisms that allow you to disconnect from external stressors and reconnect with the present and your physical self. They can include any activity that brings your attention to what's happening right now and reminds your brain that there is no immediate danger. While most people think of grounding as walking barefoot outdoors, and that is one valuable technique, the options for grounding are much broader. One of my favorite options is box breathing, shown in Image 2. Box breathing (also called square breathing) is simple and effective. Breathe in for four seconds, hold for four seconds, exhale for four seconds, hold for four seconds, and repeat. Even just two to three minutes of box breathing can dramatically increase your body's oxygen levels, calm the nervous system, and ease worry.

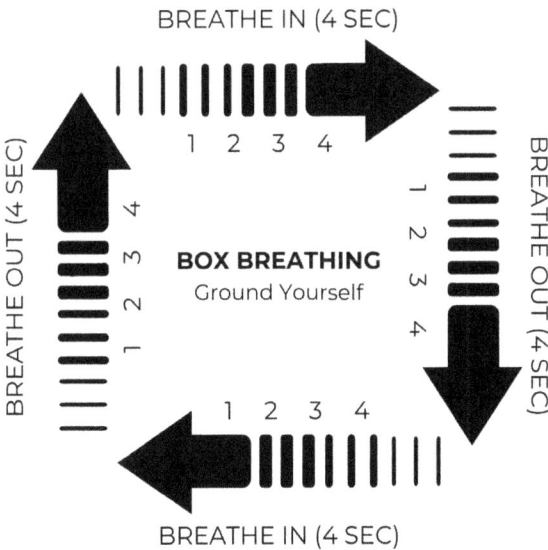

BREATHE IN (4 SEC)

BREATHE OUT (4 SEC)

BREATHE OUT (4 SEC)

BOX BREATHING
Ground Yourself

1 2 3 4

1 2 3 4

1 2 3 4

1 2 3 4

BREATHE IN (4 SEC)

Image 2

More great options for grounding include moderate sun exposure, bird watching, gardening, treading water, painting or drawing, walking on the beach, and playing a musical instrument. I recommend some form of grounding each day, if possible, but three to five times per week at a minimum.

- **Control the controllables.** Quickly evaluate the stress you're under. What do you have no control over right now? Let that go. What do you have some control over? Put that to the side for a moment. What do you have total control over? This is where you start. You typically have control over some of your inputs and outputs. What are you letting in, and what are you letting out? Control those first with about 80 percent of your energy. Then let your remaining energy shift to what you have some control over. Often, this will be aspects of your immediate environment or social setting. Put no energy at all into areas beyond your control. We will go deeper into your sphere of control later in this chapter.

- **Remember that activity reclaims agency.** Generally, the solutions to feelings of physical stress will come from mental strategies, and the solutions to feeling mental stress will come from physical activity. Often, the best solution to con-

Even just two to three minutes of box breathing can dramatically increase your body's oxygen levels, calm the nervous system, and ease worry.

suming thoughts is repetitive action. There is a reason basketball players have a routine before shooting free throws, and why golfers have a certain process for lining up a putt. The action pattern allows the brain to retreat to the safety of "been here, done this." Under stress, your brain will look for a point of focus. I can't tell you how many times, as a teacher, I spent the last few minutes before class stressing over an activity I had planned. But as soon as I stood up, walked to the door, and started welcoming students into the room, all that worry faded because it was time for action. When you feel mentally overwhelmed, revert to a familiar movement pattern. You'll be amazed at how quickly you feel back in control and able to make decisions with greater clarity and agency.

BUILDING MOMENTUM

The impact of long-term stress ripples through your intrapersonal and interpersonal relationships and, as we have seen, wreaks havoc on your physical well-being. Unaddressed stress can lead to feeling overwhelmed, socially isolated, self-defeated, and off-balance. Daily actions like those previously mentioned are great practice in minimizing the impact of stress. But to tackle long-term stress, we need to dig a bit deeper to address the root causes. This will come through a deliberate process of building up new stress-management skills. These skills will originate from an internal locus of control, then flow into new response patterns and reward systems and, ultimately, be sustained through the strength of our social connections. Visit holyfitcoaching.com/smallwins to download free resources, including a stress toolkit.

STEP 1: **Develop an internal locus of control.**

Not everything is under your control. You can't change all your circumstances or the people around you. But you do have some control. Your choices will impact your outcome, and you are not helpless or hopeless.

The Sphere of Control Model is a useful framework for managing stress by focusing on what you have control over. Here are three tips to reduce stress using this model:

- **Identify what's within your control:** Take time to reflect on your sources of stress. Make a list of the factors within your control and those outside of your control. For example, you can control your reactions, decisions, and actions, but you may not have control over external events or other people's behavior. By recognizing what you can influence, you can direct your energy toward those areas.

- **Prioritize and let go:** Once you've identified what's within your control, prioritize your efforts on the most important and manageable aspects. Often, we spread ourselves too thin by trying to control everything, which can lead to increased stress. Learn to let go of what is beyond your control, accepting that you can't change them. This shift in focus can reduce stress as you become more efficient and effective in addressing what matters most.

- **Practice mindfulness and acceptance:** Incorporate mindfulness techniques into your daily routine to help you stay present and accept situations as they are. Mindfulness can help you avoid ruminating on events outside of your control and prevent unnecessary stress. Techniques like deep breathing, meditation, and being fully engaged in the present moment can be incredibly helpful.

STEP 2: **Do the basics.**

Nothing frustrated me more as a teacher than when students would not do daily classwork and then asked for extra credit to boost their grades. I would gently (at least most of the time) remind them that extra credit has the word "extra" in it for a reason. It is in addition to, not a replacement for, their daily classwork. They needed to do the basic work assigned, and their grades would probably take care of themselves. Makes sense, right? Flip that common sense lens back to you and your actions. How much of your stress is self-induced or escalated because you are skipping over basic health habits? How often do you find yourself drawn to a novel health hack or supplementation when you haven't gotten serious about what you already know you should be doing? That hits hard.

Do the basics daily. Prioritize sleep, movement, whole foods, mindfulness, hydration, limiting alcohol, and being true to your word. The basics won't solve everything, but they certainly make it easier to identify where you need to implement more detailed steps. A foundation of compliance with your health priorities is the biggest step you can take to see a general de-escalation of self-perpetuated stress. The simple work isn't sexy. It's not flashy. But it is effective.

STEP 3: **Create social connections.**

Social connections are hard. In the modern world, many people feel alone or devoid of true connections with others. The number of our interactions with strangers at a distance is far higher than at any point in human history. At the same time, the daily interactions with close, trusted relationships are much lower than in most human societies of the past. The lack of social connection is devastating to our internal sense of well-being. When we see someone who we know and trust, serotonin is released in the brain. Serotonin makes us feel at ease and that we have enough of what we need; it can even lead to feelings of bliss and delight.

We have all experienced the pain of social loss. Being separated from our romantic partner. Sending a child to camp for the first time. The untimely death of a loved one. The discomfort of temporary loss and the pain of permanent loss are powerful indicators that we are extremely social beings. John Powell, in *The Secret of Staying in Love*, said, "It is an absolute human certainty that no one can know his own beauty or perceive a sense of his own worth until it has been reflected back to him in the mirror of another loving, caring human being." Nothing is more powerful than deep social connections to tell us that we will be okay.

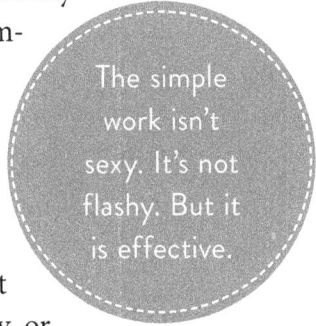

> The simple work isn't sexy. It's not flashy. But it is effective.

Invest extensively in caring relationships. It doesn't matter if it is with a pet, a romantic partner, family relationships, or friendships. Foster a sense of play, find delight in activities with others, and express human emotions face to face. This prescription is vital for each of us: You were not created to go through life alone, and you have a deep need for connection!

REMOVING OBSTACLES

Here are a few common concerns for this Hack and how to address them.

I keep getting caught in old stress response patterns. It is hard to kill off old patterns. The best strategy to help with this is called "Notice and Name." You first have to notice the old pattern. The sooner you notice yourself falling into the pattern, the better. For example, when I am stressed, I tend to lose patience when noise levels are high. With four kids in the house, the noise is always there, but my response is different under stress. So, I have to pause and notice the pattern. Then I have to name it. Naming a pattern holds power. "Oh, this is just X again." A named enemy that you've beaten before is always less scary than an unknown enemy. For me, calling out "Stressed Out Sound Sensitivity" helps me identify a known pattern and fall back on strategies I know work for me and my family.

I'm just an overthinker. High achiever, overthinker, go-getter … these are often labels we use to justify our stress and maybe even hide our stress dependency. In our society, it is entirely possible to lose the ability to relax or remember what relaxation feels like. It is likely that your sympathetic nervous system is consistently elevated. This can lead to adrenal fatigue if you do not allow your para-sympathetic nervous system to do its job. Don't let your labels keep you from being healthy in the long term. Learn to let go of your thinking and be in the moment more. Your body and loved ones will thank you.

My life is stressful, and I can't change that. No, you can't. But you can choose to use good stress to your advantage while limiting the impact of bad stress. Even with stress, you have choices and options. Who do you choose to be around? Where is your head? Are your coping mechanisms taking you somewhere, or are they contributing to the problem? Do you notice and name your stress patterns early? What can you control a bit better when under stress? Be encouraged by your growth, even when your circumstances haven't changed.

THE HACK IN ACTION

Do you remember John's story from Hack 3 and his success in changing his diet? There is more to that story that might help you understand the significance of his weight loss and lifestyle changes. Stress, stress eating, and the lack of positive social connections played a large role in his rapid weight gain and loss of confidence.

A lot of John's weight gain took place when life circumstances forced him to move in with an unsupportive and, oftentimes, toxic family member. As his mental health worsened, he felt more and more areas slip out of his control. The compounding stress of an unhealthy home environment and relational uncertainty led John to use food for comfort. Junk foods and stress eating became habitual. It did not take long for him to realize that he could not continue on like this for long.

John took action. He sacrificed time and energy to make finding a new place to live feasible. He hired a coach to help get his eating and exercise habits under control. John acted and reclaimed agency over life circumstances and stress.

John still walks several miles almost every day for his mental and physical health. He knows how valuable movement is for him to let go of stress and have a physical outlet. He is quick to notice when he is eating food out of stress and not to fuel his body. John calls out stress eating quickly and jumps into his new routines to regain control over those impulses.

The coolest part of John's story is the success he's seen, even after life led him back into the exact scenario where all his troubles began. Yes, due to a variety of circumstances, John needed to move back into that same living environment as before. But this time, he was armed and ready. John had a stronger social network around him, much better coping skills, and a commitment to protect his boundaries and priorities. The circumstances were the same; the triggers were still there. But the response patterns were a complete 180 degrees from two years prior. John's story shows the power of taming your stress and realizing that your circumstances do not have control over you or your choices.

⊩⊪

Facing and managing stressors can be an opportunity for learning, adaptation, and personal development. In moderate amounts, stress can serve as a motivational force. It can push you to work harder, stay disciplined, and achieve your fitness goals. The stress of competition, for example, can drive athletes to excel. Stress also helps with reaction and action. Stress triggers the body's fight-or-flight response, which can enhance physical performance in the short term. This can be beneficial during high-intensity workouts or athletic competitions. But you can't stay there. Instead, it's crucial to combine stress reduction with effective stress management strategies, such as problem-solving, seeking support, and practicing self-care, to achieve lasting well-being and resilience in the face of life's most stressful moments.

DON'T WAIT TO BE MOTIVATED

Keep Going Even When You Don't See Results

*We must lay before him what
is in us, not what ought to be in us.*
— C.S. LEWIS, AUTHOR AND THEOLOGIAN

THE PROBLEM: WE EXPECT THE FEELING TO COME BEFORE THE ACTION

YOU'VE BEEN HERE before—sitting on the couch, scrolling through social media, or staring at a blank page, waiting to feel "motivated." But what does that mean? What finally compels us, if ever, to get up and do what needs to be done? We tell ourselves that we'll start that new project, hit the gym, or finally clean out the cluttered garage as soon as motivation magically appears. But here's the truth: motivation is a myth.

I don't mean that motivation doesn't exist. I mean that the modern understanding of motivation as some feeling that acts as the primary force behind our actions is false. Dictionaries define motivation as "the process or act of motivating." I don't know about you, but that isn't helpful in painting a clear picture of what motivation is or how it works. We sit and wonder why we are not doing the things we know we need to do. We wait for an impulse or inspiration. We consume more content and information. We have the ideas but not the follow-through.

You believe that the reason you aren't acting is that you don't care enough. "If I really cared about it, I would act." So you exert energy in trying to make yourself care more. But that is backward. You wouldn't be reading this book if you didn't care about your health and want to find lasting change. Waiting to "care enough" turns a physical action into mental friction. Waiting for motivation is the widest path to procrastination. You've created a mental bookmark, which is basically telling your brain that you need to revisit this idea over and over. Mental bookmarks are useful for big decisions. It's similar to saving a resource you will need to reference often during a large project. But you may be using them for small decisions, in-the-moment choices, and tasks that could easily be routines.

Let me illustrate. Imagine bookmarking the idea "I need to eat healthier." It's a great idea at first glance. But if you eat three to five times a day and revisit that thought with every meal or snack, that is twenty-one to thirty times per week that you are thinking about what you need to do *instead of doing it*. You haven't taken any specific action to solve the problem but have put the problem front and center on an endless loop. Amplify that analogy across all the habits or choices you are actively trying to change. It is no wonder that your brain is overloaded with bookmarks and feels overwhelmed trying to keep them all open and organized.

Waiting on motivation is selective de-motivation. I could survey your life and find many areas where you are highly motivated. I also bet that you never sat around waiting to be motivated in those areas. Every attempt to motivate yourself to "care enough" will only feed feelings of guilt, frustration, and insufficiency. Your problem is not that you don't care enough. Your problem is not that you need more evidence or proof that your health matters. Your problem is not that you are an unmotivated person. It is that you are building mental pressure around physical problems.

You do not lack motivation. And motivation isn't good by default. We must unlearn the motivation that took us off-target and build new motivations. Every choice, even one that works against our best interest, is motivated. You have decided that the choices you make and the routines you follow are worth continuing over the cost of learning new ones. We might not be aware of the motivation, but it is there. We cannot rely on impulse when we are trying to create routines. We cannot expect the feeling to come before taking action.

THE HACK: DON'T WAIT TO BE MOTIVATED

You do not need motivation to start. Often, motivation only comes long after we've taken the first step. Think about it: Have you ever regretted going to the gym or starting a project? Probably not. But have you ever talked yourself out of starting or even lacing up your gym shoes? Of course you have. If your brain got you into a mess, don't expect that same brain to get you out of it. Action breeds motivation. Once you begin, you build momentum through small wins, and that momentum generates motivation.

We are often willing to deceive ourselves in order to cope with uncomfortable truths or situations. Psychologists call this tendency "self-deception." Numerous great works of literature, from *The Great Gatsby* to *Anna Karenina*, deal with this theme of creating comforting lies to escape uncomfortable realities. If we convince ourselves that we have a problem or a condition, we can avoid confronting the real issues of why we aren't acting the way we want to act. Waiting for the perfect time or the right dose of motivation is a form of self-deception. The great Russian novelist Ivan Turgenev put it this way: "If we wait for the moment when everything, absolutely everything is ready, we shall never begin." Messy action will always beat perfect procrastination.

It's easy to say you are waiting to be motivated. Feeling motivated (or not feeling it) is in the mind. It's vague. Practicing an action is in the present. It's practical. When we are afraid of taking the first step, we tend to default to the safety of our excuses. But that is covering the deeper issue with a layer of denial. The solution is to just act. Instead of waiting, move. Remember: if you acted on it, you would care about it. Doing the thing is what makes you want to do the thing. Doing the thing is what gives you the skills you need to keep doing the thing. Feeling motivated is great when it is present, but consistency of action is where success is nurtured.

Success in any endeavor is the result of consistent effort, not sporadic bursts of motivation. Those who achieve greatness do so because they show up and put in the work, whether they feel motivated or not. Consistency builds habits and routines, which are the foundation of progress. When you consistently work toward your goals, you create a pattern of behavior that becomes ingrained in your daily life. This habitual approach makes it easier to stay on track, even when you don't feel particularly motivated.

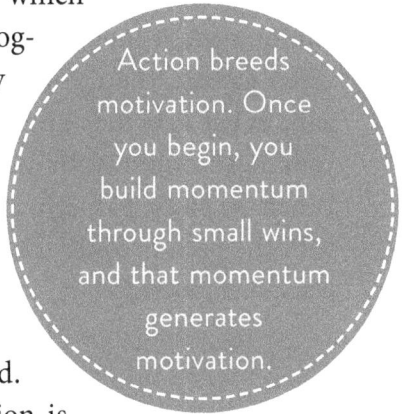

> Action breeds motivation. Once you begin, you build momentum through small wins, and that momentum generates motivation.

Let's reframe what motivation is. A more practical definition is that motivation is a continued choice to pursue one course of action by forgoing the alternatives. As author and thinker Steven Pressfield said, "At some point, the pain of not doing it becomes greater than the pain of doing it." When that pain becomes great enough, you will choose to pursue a better route. The empowering truth of this concept is that you are capable of making that decision at any moment, not only after the pain becomes unbearable. Expect motivation to fade and anticipate how you will choose to continue. You will never sit around waiting to be motivated when you know that motivation is simply the outcome of your choices.

That means it is essential to be incredibly selective in what you say yes to. I know I have an addictive personality. When I get into a new hobby or interest, it can easily consume my thoughts and attention. I enjoyed playing video games when I was younger, but there came a point in my midtwenties when I knew they were a distraction for me. Losing sleep, losing time to read, and losing time with my family made it too costly to continue investing time into video games. The framework I like to use is head/heart/will. What activities and choices in front of you activate your head, ignite your heart, and align with your will? When we swap fear, ego, and impulse for head, heart, and will, the path becomes clear and motivation flows from a place of abundance!

WHAT YOU CAN DO TOMORROW

- **Remember to ask what the healthier version of you would do right now.** We can ask ourselves that question to find the practical steps we know will benefit us the most. As we discussed in Hack 4, when we defer to a future, healthier version of ourselves, we can think outside of the present moment. We can spot the patterns and bigger picture a bit easier with less of our ego at stake. Let's say you would like to stick to mindful, balanced eating while traveling. Knowing which restaurants or snacks the healthier version of you would pick will help you zoom out and see the full landscape. You can use this concept in multiple ways. You can ask yourself, "Who would the healthier version of me surround myself with?" to help identify healthy relationships. And "How long would the healthier version of me press on?" when you want to quit. When you know what your healthier self would do, you can predict what choices now will make you most proud later. That's a permission slip to get out of your head and act.

- **Find your "why."** The "why" sentiment still holds value when it comes to motivation. Your why is shorthand for the core truths and principles that shape your purpose. I like to think of motivation as the fusion of knowledge and purpose. You have a much deeper reserve to pull from when your path is clearly linked to your why. This is particularly important when life gets tough. Let's go back to the goal of eating better while traveling: Why do you want to eat better during this trip? Is it because you want to keep your gut happy, have more energy for fun activities, and feel proud of your choices? Having clarity always helps. Sticking to the course feels easy when life is easy, but without a deeper sense of purpose, we will fade off under pressure.

- **Be aware of trials and tradeoffs.** We were far more likely to give something a try when we were children. Most things were new to us, and we weren't self-conscious about trying and failing. But then middle school came along. Often, we became self-conscious and concerned that everyone was watching us.

    I remember a middle school swing dance event where I built up the courage to ask a girl to dance and then abandoned her halfway into the song. The girl I ditched that day is now my wife of almost fifteen years (I'm pretty sure she has forgiven me by now). As I matured a bit and entered my senior year in high school, I realized that I cared a heck of a lot more about what she thought than what anyone else thought. I knew I needed to step up and try again. Life is about trials and tradeoffs. I had to trade the fear of rejection and embarrassment for the courage to ask her to go out with me. Hannah was the first girl I ever asked out, and now I can't imagine my life without her.

    Maybe you tried and failed before. Maybe you lacked the skills or courage last time. Don't let that one mistake burn you twice by keeping you from trying again someday. I have many, many clients who come to me so accustomed to eating highly processed foods that they can't imagine life without fast food and junk food. Over time, their meals become more balanced, and their snack choices improve. Inevitably, they report feeling awful and physically worse anytime they drop back into their old eating patterns. They see that the swap for better food makes them feel better. Once you know the tradeoff is worth it, it is far more likely that you will consistently make the same choices and push past the fear of failure.

• **Ask yourself, "If this, then ...."** It's great to know your purpose and goals, but what do you do when you feel overwhelmed by the number of options available to pursue? This is one of my favorite mental frames for deciding on a course of action. If this is my goal, what daily actions do I need to do to get me there? My goal is to eat better on the road. So what steps do I need to think through to make this happen? I could keep high-protein breakfast options in the hotel fridge and stock my vehicle or day bag with high-quality, shelf-stable snacks. Now I have some clear action steps. Here are a couple more examples of how to state this frame: If this is my purpose, then what thoughts and actions will best help me fulfill that purpose? If this is the kind of person I want to be, then who can I surround myself with to push me in that direction? Using this strategy will help isolate the most logical next steps in light of where you currently are and the direction in which you hope to move.

- **Deploy an "advance team."** You can know what to do, but if you put so many hurdles in the way, that momentum is almost impossible to maintain. Or you can clear the path in advance. Don't wander into the wilderness without a scout party and advance preparation. A scout party ventures into the unknown, identifies potential obstacles, and gathers crucial information about the terrain. Similarly, when trying to establish better habits, your "advance team" could be your own research and planning. Advance teams make the path more accessible, removing barriers that might slow you down. In your habit-building journey, this corresponds to eliminating barriers and temptations. Arrange your environment to make it easier to engage in your desired habits.

For example, remove unhealthy snacks from your pantry if you're trying to eat better. The advance team leaves markers and signs along the trail, guiding you in the right direction. They ensure you stay on track and don't get lost. Similarly, establish clear reminders and cues for your desired habits. Set alarms, create to-do lists, or place visual cues in your environment to prompt you to take action. In this analogy, the "advance team" represents the proactive approach of preparation, planning, and support that can make establishing and sustaining better habits a smoother and more successful journey.

If this is the kind of person I want to be, then who can I surround myself with to push me in that direction?

BUILDING MOMENTUM

Discipline is the starting line. As adherence builds, momentum follows. With more momentum comes the repetitions needed to develop lasting habits. And, as we have seen, lasting habits are where real results happen. It's easy to look at others further along the path than us and think they have some secret that propelled them ahead. But the secret is that they have been practicing certain habits for years, and you're just starting. This Chinese proverb rings true: "The best time to plant a tree was twenty years ago. The second best time is now." You cannot let the absence of current results prevent you from taking the necessary steps to get future results. There are no shortcuts. There is only building new patterns, breaking old patterns, learning new habits, unlearning old habits, and stepping out in faith and hope when things feel scary.

STEP 1: **Build consistency through new habits.**

Habits can stay with you forever. The neurological pathways that are created with repeated patterns never dissolve. This means bad habits can stick around forever, and so can good habits.

The trick is to feed new good habits and starve old bad habits. Let's break that down together. Habits operate in three stages: trigger, process, and reward (see Image 3). The *trigger* is the signal that activates an ingrained process (think the bell in Pavlov's dog experiment). The *process* is the instinctive pattern of thoughts and actions that follows the trigger (the dogs salivate when they hear the bell due to their conditioning). The *reward* is the validation (either through intrinsic or extrinsic signals) your brain gets when it completes the process as programmed.

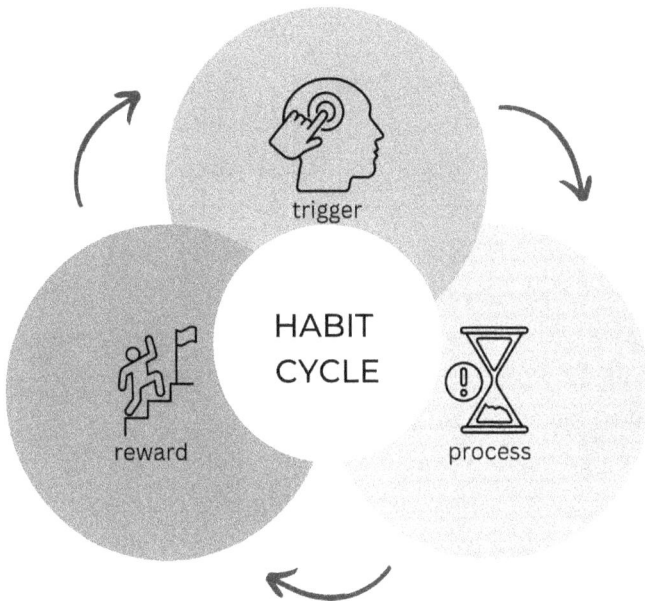

Image 3

You can pinpoint naturally occurring triggers to build your process and reward. For example, your alarm goes off each morning. Your process right now is probably to hit snooze (maybe multiple times, if we're honest). The reward is getting to sleep a bit more. We can swap that. When your alarm goes off, practice turning off the alarm and getting up without hitting snooze. Now you have to reward the action. Maybe you spend two minutes deep breathing, five minutes in prayer or mindfulness, or you drink a glass of water. A simple reward will go a long way in making it easier to be more intentional. This is why I focus on celebrating small wins. What you celebrate, you will see more of in your life. But maximize the rewards for new habits that you want to build and strengthen.

STEP 2: Unlearn habits.

Somewhere along the journey of adulthood, we forget that habits can be unlearned. Yes, habits stick around in our systems, but old habits can fade if they aren't reinforced for an extended period. I love this analogy from author and philosopher G.K. Chesterton: "Fairy tales do not tell children the dragons exist. Children already know that dragons exist. Fairy tales tell children the dragons can be killed." We need to remember that the strongholds we want to be rid of can be toppled.

Let's go back to trigger, process, and reward. How do we unlearn an ingrained habit? Which part of the pattern can we change most easily? The trigger is often out of our control. If another driver cuts you off on the highway, you can't control that. Well, what about our reactions—the process? The process usually happens too quickly for us to stop it. You get road rage and do or say something out of anger in direct response. The reward is different. The reward isn't automated. In the case of road rage, the reward will come when you validate and justify your behavior because the other driver is obviously incompetent.

You can choose not to follow through with the reward. You can instead be honest with yourself and even create a non-reward response (for example, you have to drive 1 mph under the speed limit for three miles). By refusing to reward the habit, over time, your brain will stop reinforcing the process. The reward is the hit of dopamine, the sense of accomplishment or completion. Without that sensation, you will no longer see the benefit of following through on the process. Maybe you had a tough day at work. Your natural response is to want to let off some steam, and your favorite show is just the distraction you need. But then one episode isn't enough. You feel you "deserve" to binge-watch one more TV episode and sacrifice sleep. Realize that this "reward" has a cost and might lead to more stress tomorrow. Be careful what you reward. Rewarded habits get stronger over time. Find ways to deny the reward for habits you want to end.

STEP 3: Take the leap.

My wife says I like sad movies. I tell her they aren't sad, just melancholic (which basically means sad). I like sad music too. The band Switchfoot sings a great song that I could listen to on repeat, and it's called "The Blues." The main lyric in the chorus impacted me as a young teen. I remember listening to it on my MP3 player in the car while holding a cloth to my eyebrow on the way to get stitches from a tough run-in with a metal post while playing basketball. The song is about how any day could be the day everything falls apart. It hit me then that you never know what can happen by the end of the day. If you listen to the song, you may think it's a bit depressing but may also realize that it's true. You never know what the day holds, good or bad. It may be a day when you start down a new path that dramatically alters your future in incredible ways.

At the time of this writing, it was about three years ago when I thought I could be successful as a fitness and nutrition coach. It was just a regular day. But that thought was the seed I planted and watered. Then I had to cultivate the idea and take action on it. Now my life is completely different, my career has diverged from what I had planned, and I can have an impact on thousands of individuals. What seeds are you planting? Be careful what you plant because you will reap what you sow. It will be a day like this one when your life starts to change. Do your best to make sure that change is for the good.

STEP 4: Build routines and rituals.

Your brain can do two things really well: routine and ritual. I like to think of routine as the patterns that feel easy to repeat because the brain recognizes the next step. Every system we build as humans has routine built in, either intentionally or unintentionally. We fall into routines quickly. Routines come naturally, but we are not accustomed to building them intentionally in our personal lives. The best way to start is to understand the sequence of duration, path, and outcome.

Neuroscientist Dr. Andrew Huberman often talks about duration, path, and outcome. In simple terms, we are asking, *What am I doing? Where am I going? And what's the point?* Every routine provides answers to those three questions. The cool thing is that we can use this sequence to build new routines. As much as you might be tempted to, don't start with high-level tasks. The amount of focus and thought to create a routine around a five-year plan, for example, is incredibly high. The best place to start is with activities that are low in duration, path, and outcome, and then build from there. We already discussed setting a bedtime routine. That is a great example of a low duration, path, and outcome. But let's look at a more extended routine: a monthly personal fitness assessment.

MONTHLY FITNESS ASSESSMENT		
Measure →	Reflect →	Set Goals
Duration: 15 minutes (on the first day of each month) Path: Fitness Progress and Goal-Setting		
• Measure relevant fitness metrics (e.g., weight, body measurements, progress photos, or fitness test results).	• Reflect on your fitness achievements and challenges for 10 minutes.	• Set new fitness goals or adjust existing ones for the next month for 5 minutes.
Outcome: You have a clear view of your progress, celebrate your accomplishments, and have realistic goals for continuous improvement.		

Ritual is different. Ritual is best understood as reflexive actions. What actions do you perform without thinking about them (like scratching a mosquito bite while half-asleep)? We all have small, subtle rituals associated with almost every step of our routines. They can be hard to identify, but if you were a fly on the wall, you would spot them. Being aware of these subtle signals is called interoceptive awareness. Being aware of what you do before you perform a habit can give you interesting feedback. If you have a spouse, kids, or a roommate, ask them about the things you do that you don't realize you're doing. You might be surprised by what micro-actions you do repeatedly without being aware of them. Knowledge *of* knowledge is powerful. Sometimes, you can change or be more conscious of an entire routine or action pattern just by taking notice of your rituals.

REMOVING OBSTACLES

Here are a few common concerns for this Hack and how to address them.

I start a lot of things well but don't see them through. Have you ever worked for someone who would present half-baked ideas, get employees scrambling to implement the ideas, and then pull the rug out from under the initiative? How frustrating would it be to work for a boss or company that did that on an endless loop? That's what your body has to endure while listening to your brain. It can seem directionless, start/stop, and in a constant state of confusion. That's not where you want to be. Fire your CEO! You don't have to go so far as writing a letter of termination (although you could), but anytime you want to jump into something new without thinking it through, remind yourself that it is the old CEO talking, and they aren't in charge anymore. The new CEO is more intentional, forward-thinking, and likely to stick to the game plan.

I want to change, but my current routines are comforting. The hard truth is that you're not in enough pain yet. The comfort of your current situation may deter you from making a change, even if what you're doing now is not fulfilling. You may not believe that change is necessary yet. But play it out. Where is your current trajectory taking you? Where will you be two years from now? Five years? Ten years? Maybe you need to come back five years from now when the discomfort of your current situation is so great that you can't ignore it. I hope you don't. I hope you make the changes now and never experience that unnecessary pain. Don't trade lasting happiness for momentary pleasure and comfort.

I'm not sure the timing is right to make a lot of changes. Waiting for the right timing is the same as waiting for motivation. When you get into a holding pattern, you get complacent. You can get to a place where, even when the timing *is* right, you have zero momentum and miss the moment. Imagine your car is running poorly, but you're busy and it doesn't seem that serious, so you put off taking it to the shop. What could have been a quick fix ends up becoming a major repair, and your car has to be towed to the mechanic. You end up spending more time and money by delaying the repair than you ever would have spent if you had put a little time into upkeep and maintenance. Make small adjustments along the way before the choice is out of your hands.

What if I lose friendships or relationships when I change my habits and routines? Imagining how people will respond when you change your lifestyle is problematic, at best. You have no idea what they are thinking about you now, much less what they might think about you later. For all you know, they already wish you had made these changes. Your fear is a projection of loss aversion. We resist change so much that we invent hypothetical losses to convince ourselves we are better off staying put. But what if your fears come true? If you lose friends or relationships because you are stepping into a healthier version of yourself, then will you actually miss those relationships in the long run? If the people surrounding you are not in favor of you being healthier, happier, and around longer, then losing them might be an additional benefit.

THE HACK IN ACTION

I felt trapped. I was teaching in a school that left me drained daily, and our family was struggling financially in major ways. It was winter 2020, and pandemic teaching and coaching had me on empty. I thought I had found the way out. My master's degree is in Russian and East European Studies. I made it to the final interview stage to be the regional director of a large international organization that does humanitarian work in Eastern Europe and Central Asia.

I had the language, degree, and international experience. But the organization decided to hire the other finalist candidate. It is hard to describe the sinking feeling, the pit in my stomach, when I got that phone call. I was devastated and immediately dreading the remainder of the school year. I had my faith but no joy. I had my family but felt insufficient to lead well. I had a career but no direction.

I saw a couple of fit teacher friends on social media doing online fitness coaching. I had no idea that was a thing, but one of those teachers ended up leaving her teaching position to coach full time. I thought, "Maybe I could do that." I thought I could make enough income by coaching online as a side gig to make ends meet. So I jumped in. We went further into debt so that I could hire a business mentor and do things the right way. It was scary, and I am not 100 percent sure my wife believed in the idea, but she did believe in me.

My experience as an educator, writer, and leader, plus my passion for fitness and my willingness to do what it took, combined beautifully to help me get clients. I realized I had a perspective that people responded to, and my early clients started getting results. Within nine months, I decided not to renew my teaching contract. One week after I submitted my resignation, Hannah and I were shocked to find out that we were expecting our fourth child. Talk about another moment of deep doubt. I remember telling my wife's family on April 2 that I was not returning to teaching the following year. My father-in-law looked directly at me and asked me if that was a late April Fool's joke. Part of me wanted to say "Yes, sir" and ask for my teaching job back.

But here I am. My family, in-laws (yes, even my father-in-law), friends, and other fitness professionals have supported and encouraged me every step of the way. My passion for helping others who feel stuck comes from that core memory of how I felt during that pivotal moment in my life. Helping even one person not to feel that sense of uncertainty lights a fire in me. My message to you is to do the scary thing. Jump in. Even if you don't know the second step, you know the first one. Take the step that is in front of you. You know what it feels like to be where you are now. But you have no idea what you will feel or experience when you step out and do hard things.

‖┣━┫‖

Waiting on motivation is a fool's game. If you want to accomplish your goals and make meaningful progress, don't rely on motivation to get you started. Instead, embrace discipline, create routines, set deadlines, and take that first step. Remember, action precedes motivation, and success is the reward for consistent effort. You may have heard the saying, "Don't be upset by the results you didn't get with the work you didn't do." Put in the work and see what happens. You will never regret the effort you put into the pursuits that light you up!

LOVE WHAT YOUR BODY CAN DO

Help Your Body Function at Its Best

*The way to love anything is
to realize that it may be lost.*
— G.K. CHESTERTON, AUTHOR AND PHILOSOPHER

THE PROBLEM: WE ARE CONSTANTLY TOLD OUR BODIES ARE BROKEN

THE CLASSIC CHILDREN'S book *The Phantom Toll-booth* by Norton Juster includes a powerful analogy about being careful what you turn to for solutions. In this whimsical tale, a boy named Milo and his friends take a bizarre journey to an imaginary world, where they have a peculiar dinner. The first course was soup, and the more they ate, the hungrier they became. Bowl after bowl, Milo and his friends continued to get hungrier and hungrier.

Their host remarked how they must have been very full to have needed so many bowls of subtraction soup.

The concept of subtraction soup can remind us how easily we focus our energy on solutions that actually make the problems worse, particularly when it comes to our health.

Unfortunately, the current state of the health and fitness industry, heavily influenced by social media, has fostered a widespread culture of misinformation, unrealistic standards, and harmful advice. One of the most glaring issues is the prevalence of unqualified individuals offering health and fitness advice. Influencers with no formal training or certification often promote unverified dietary plans, exercise routines, and even supplements with clear profit and personal brand incentives. This can mislead vulnerable individuals, particularly impressionable teens, and jeopardize their physical and mental well-being.

Cambridge University Press published research by E. Byrne, J. Kearney, and C. MacEvilly titled "The Role of Influencer Marketing and Social Influencers in Public Health" (2017), and it discussed the problem, saying, "Many influencers are not registered dietitians or qualified nutritionists and often share false or misleading nutritional information with no scientific evidence; this can negatively impact diet and health. ... Registered dietitians and qualified nutritionists are the best source of credible, accurate nutrition information."

Moreover, social media perpetuates the myth of the "perfect" body, leading to ever-increasing body image issues, low self-esteem, and eating disorders. The constant stream of edited and filtered images can distort reality, making many feel inadequate and unworthy. The pursuit of likes, follows, and engagement has led to dangerous behaviors, including extreme dieting, harmful detoxes, high-risk exercise, and reliance on performance-enhancing substances. These shortcuts often result in adverse health effects, and they set unrealistic expectations.

We are constantly told that our bodies are broken and that certain supplements, products, exercises, diets, or new approaches will "fix" us. I am a firm believer in taking action to see self-improvement, but the grift culture has severely muddied the waters on what truly sustainable health looks like. The basics aren't sexy. First, principles don't sell courses or memberships. Simple, whole foods don't make supplement companies and their paid promoters millions of dollars. Moderation and mindfulness won't line the pockets of for-profit public health institutions. All the quick fixes and fitness fads in the world will not change the health crisis we are facing. They will only keep people feeling overwhelmed, disillusioned, and frustrated that another attempt didn't solve the problem.

You don't lose your health, energy, or sex drive overnight. It's a slow fade. You wake up one morning, and you don't like how you feel, look, or act. What took a moment to realize actually took years of built-up poor choices. Have you ever had debts pile up so much that paying just the interest became a challenge? It wasn't one purchase that caused the problem. It was a pattern of decisions or inattentiveness to bills and debts. The compounding interest builds on itself until what was once a simple payment becomes impossible to manage.

Unhealthy choices are like bad debts. Your body isn't worse at healing itself than when you were younger. It's that the accumulation of "bad debts" has built to a level that it can't handle paying off the interest. Just because you didn't see the effects doesn't mean they weren't there. The accumulation of junk and debt from poor choices will catch up. A month or two of better choices won't make things better. A pill, a crash diet, and a few intense workouts won't repair the effects of years of neglect.

THE HACK: LOVE WHAT YOUR BODY CAN DO

Our bodies aren't broken. Our bodies are fearfully and wonderfully made. Even if a certain aspect of your health or body is not where you would like it to be, there are so many things your body is doing well to keep you functioning. The more I study the human body, the more amazed I am at its ability to adapt. Our bodies are incredibly responsive to our environment and inputs to protect, correct, and filter. Love what your body can do, and don't take it for granted.

Balancing an appreciation of what our bodies can do with a desire to improve can be a challenge. I recently told my oldest son that we would start biking trails together. He is almost twelve years old, smart and creative, and he isn't interested in team sports like his brothers. I wanted to find more ways to spend time outdoors with him. We went riding in our neighborhood to get some practice in before finding longer trails. We started riding up the biggest hill in the subdivision. He got about halfway up the hill and then got off his seat and began walking the bike up the hill. I challenged him to try to ride all the way to the top.

His immediate reaction was to say it was too hard. But I encouraged him that he could do it and that this would help him be stronger for our longer rides coming up. He adjusted his gears, got back on the seat, and made it all the way to the top!

The easiest path does not go to the top of the mountain. Embrace the hard path if you are looking for a body, mindset, and resilience that few can achieve. Embracing hard doesn't mean the same thing as putting undue pressure on your mind or systems. Changing your body will take longer than you think it will. Work hard, be patient, and have fun with it. Your body already knows how to do many things well. Let it do its job by staying out of the way most of the time, changing your activity outputs some of the time, and being mindful about what you put in it all of the time.

Take the pressure off your body. Take the pressure off how much you think you should weigh or how you look in the mirror. No one will love you more if you're skinnier. But they might get to love you longer if you're healthier. In his book *Tiny Habits*, author BJ Fogg issues an important challenge: "Write this phrase on a small piece of paper: I change best by feeling good, not by feeling bad." Pressure, guilt, and comparison will never make you feel your best. And if you don't feel your best, how will you ever change to become your best?

Stop being robbed of enjoying the present because your future health seems so uncertain.

Start with simple habits today that will make tomorrow easier and give you hope for the future. Control the controllables. Let go of what gives you pressure and increase what you protect!

WHAT YOU CAN DO TOMORROW

- **Protect your gut.** Sit down to eat at least one to two meals per day. Slow down. Chew food thoroughly with meals, even if it makes mealtimes take longer. Digestion starts with chewing. If you are inhaling food, it's going to cause additional discomfort and bloating. Think about meal timing as a gut health strategy by keeping meals three to four hours apart. Keep snacks at least one hour before or after a meal. Look at fiber and fiber sources.

  Soluble fiber helps regulate blood sugar by slowing the absorption of carbs, and it helps lower fats in the blood. It keeps you fuller longer because of the slower absorption, and it also feeds the good bacteria in the gut. Great examples are fruit, veggies, beans, and seeds.

  Insoluble fiber helps your body process waste, improves digestion, and reduces constipation. Great examples are bran, husks of whole grains, nuts, seeds, oats, brown rice, green beans, raspberries, kidney beans, cauliflower, peas, potatoes, leafy veggies, whole wheat bread, and rice.

- **Protect your immune system.** Consume a variety of fruits and vegetables rich in vitamins, minerals, and antioxidants. Sleep seven to nine hours per night as often as possible. Take daily movement breaks. Carry a reusable water bottle to remind yourself to stay hydrated. Take a daily vitamin. Wash your hands regularly. And maintain strong, close social connections. All this sounds basic, but remember that the basics are effective.

- **Protect your bones.** Resistance training is the number one way to build stronger joints, ligaments, tendons, and bones. Resistance bands, weight machines, free weights, and even body-weight exercises are incredibly effective at protecting and increasing overall joint and bone health. Within resistance training, compound exercises are the absolute best way to change your muscular health. Any exercise that uses more than one muscle group to complete a repetition is a compound movement. You not only burn calories, but you also address coordination, strength, mobility, and flexibility issues that go unaddressed by most cardio activities. Bravely embrace these movements and lifts. You can start light, get a solid foundation with your form, and then slowly build up over time. You will see incredible benefits! Examples of compound lifts are squats, push-ups, shoulder presses, bench presses, forward lunges, bent-over rows, pull-ups, and hip thrusts. Visit holyfitcoaching.com/smallwins for full how-to guides on these movements.

- **Protect your hormones.** Producing hormones requires energy. The better balanced your nutrition, the better resources your body will have to keep your hormones balanced. Eat enough calories and nutrients for your body and activity levels. The body protects reproduction first when it senses things are out of whack. When calories and nutrients are too low, the body will act quickly to down-regulate sex hormones because it senses you do not have enough intake to support new life. In women, progesterone goes first. In men, testosterone goes first. So, don't undereat or eat a deficient diet.

- **Eat healthy fats.** Much of your hormone production and brain balance is powered by fats. Eat lean proteins. Eating close to your body weight in grams of protein daily (.6 to .8 grams per pound of body weight is a solid range for most people) is a simple target to set up. Remember to activate your parasympathetic system daily to help reduce stress levels. If your stress levels are too high or your nutrient intake is too low, hormone production is one of the first systems to be impacted. Life gets harder when your hormones are out of balance.

- **Protect your soul.** I was raised to believe that we have a larger purpose than to be born, live, and die. I still believe that each of us was created in the image of God and was given a soul that will live forever. Our minds and spirits are just as important to our health as our physical state. Theologian and philosopher Augustine of Hippo said, "Care for your body as though you were going to live forever. Care for your soul as if you were going to die tomorrow." We know our bodies will eventually fail us, so make sure to invest in things that last after we are gone. Explore opportunities to invest in relationships, legacies, and making the world better for future generations.

> Start with simple habits today that will make tomorrow easier and give you hope for the future.

BUILDING MOMENTUM

What changes you isn't the result, it is the process. Some days, I still see the old me when I look in the mirror. I don't see any difference from how I looked in college or as a young dad. If you could snap your fingers and look exactly how you wanted to look right away, all your insecurities would still be there. They have a way of resurfacing, don't they?

But the work you put in? That work grounds you in your new reality. When everything is in doubt, you can look at yourself and say, "I'm different now than I was because my choices are different now than they were." It was never easy. It was never convenient. It was never perfect. But dang, it's fun! And it's rewarding, and it's worth it. And that's when you will see the new you emerge.

STEP 1: **Break the approval-seeking cycle.**

Face it: doing what is good for your health may be labeled "weird." Some parts of modern society will call you toxic or a buzz kill. I've seen adults label parents selfish for taking time alone to work out. Coworkers might call you extreme for making basic lifestyle changes. Post one photo showing you doing something positive for your body, and a long-lost cousin will call you self-obsessed. Everyone has an opinion of what they think normal is, and you cannot please everyone. Here's what you need to do: love 'em but don't listen to 'em. They aren't looking for your validation to continue their self-destructive habits, so don't look for their validation to continue your self-care efforts. The right process, the one that works for you, starts with you. It starts when you say "enough is enough" and take full responsibility and make the commitment to learn. I won't lie to you: it's a hard road. It's hard to wake up every day and be honest with yourself. You will hit hurdles, days when it feels hopeless, and moments when stress tells you to wallow in self-pity and give in to your every desire. But where will you end up if you quit then? Worse than when you started, or constantly fighting the same battles over and over. That's the truth.

STEP 2: Break the quick-fix cycle.

Imagine if a slick talker in a fancy suit told you he would increase your financial investments by 200 percent in a year at absolutely zero risk to you. You would be skeptical, and rightfully so. Let's say he shows you screenshots of dozens of clients making massive returns. He sends you video after video of those clients talking about how life-changing these returns were for them. The social proof makes you inclined to listen a bit more. Then you see a social media post from a name you've heard of endorsing this as a viable investment. Maybe you decide to invest; maybe you don't. But two years later, the entire venture is exposed as a Ponzi scheme, and millions of people lost all their investments. Everyone knew it was too good to be true, but the social evidence was compelling. This scenario is happening hundreds of thousands of times per day in the health and fitness space. Products, programs, promises, and "proof."

You're bombarded with these products and promises, but you're not being educated. You do not need vibrating waist slimmers. You do not need "Thirty Days to Trim" programs. You do not need core circuits to "tone" your abs or "flatten" your belly. You do not need a specific diet, drink, shake, or pill to "burn tummy fat fast." What you need is to embrace the slow, steady path of daily improvement. Before you ever say yes to any pitch, you need to ask why. Why do I even want visible results? Why does this proof sound so good? Am I allowing insecurities to make me vulnerable to "easy, quick fixes"? Or am I committed to my long-term health, well-being, and longevity? Am I willing to commit to lifestyle changes to be a better me? Am I going to put in the work it takes to treat my body well? Remember that being more fit is not about how you look. That can be a potential bonus, but the real benefits are almost always unseen.

STEP 3: Break the guilt cycle.

You do not have to feel guilty doing and eating what you love. Stay with me. Guilt is based on assumptions that you have acquired over your life about what is and isn't good food or good exercise. Why do you think your assumptions are correct? Because you don't remember learning them. Therefore, you again assume your beliefs must be a truth or fact that "everyone knows." But that doesn't mean you know how your body functions, how to train, or how to sustain a proper nutrition approach that feels empowering and not defeating. I do not enjoy distance running. I still do it from time to time, but I am not going to guilt myself into running long distances when I know I will not stick to it. I am better off going for walks and doing hill sprints for my cardio since I enjoy those options. The same goes for food. Why would you build guilt and derogatory labels around foods that you know you love and want to enjoy from time to time? There is a lot of wisdom in including those foods into your plan in a moderate amount.

STEP 4: **Break the generational cycle.**

We cannot change the genetic code that was passed down to us. We cannot go back and change what our home life was like as children. But we do have agency now. We have options for new choices, therapy, support systems, and habits. You can stop generational health problems in their tracks. You can. It's not easy, but you can replace the harmful or less than ideal micro-habits that you accepted as a child. The habits you create today will reverberate long after you are gone. I want my sons to have more health freedom and an easier path to sustainable habits from following my and my wife's example. Even if your children are grown or you do not have kids, a younger generation is looking up to you and can benefit from seeing how you approach your health. Be the difference maker.

STEP 5: **Break the restrictive cycle.**

Being healthier is not about removing sources of joy from your life. It's about embracing, balancing, and increasing all the things that will help you have more joy for longer. Aren't you tired of restricting? Tired of the yo-yo of cutting out foods only to rebound hard? Tired of feeling mentally beaten up by all the items and habits you are supposed to eliminate? You've tried the "less, less, less" route. It doesn't work for most people. How about embracing more? More quality food, more movement, more strength, and more vigor and energy. Do not cut out a source of joy until you have a replacement of equal or greater value built up to replace it. The curious thing is that what you once found tedious can become highly valued when it is in service of an ever-increasing source of happiness and joy.

REMOVING OBSTACLES

Here are a few common concerns for this Hack and how to address them.

I have a chronic or genetic condition that limits me. We tend to fixate on our limiting factors and allow them to dissuade us from stepping into what we can do. Whatever condition you are living with is a limitation, but you do not need to let it stop you in every avenue of life. You navigate, adjust, and find workarounds in the areas you value most. Your body deserves that same resourcefulness. I have worked with many folks who deal with chronic conditions, and with every challenge, we can take steps forward. Find someone who has had it worse but has done it better. Model after them or try to have them give you a road map. Care and protect your health to the best of your ability out of gratitude for what you can do and not out of frustration over what you can't do. No one is telling you the path will be easy. I'm here to say that the path is possible. Consult with your healthcare provider on what is appropriate for you, and take the challenge head-on!

I've tried the slow and steady route, and I end up frustrated. I've worked with people who began making great changes to their habits and nutrition, feeling more energized, mentally stable, confident, and in control, but they were still frustrated. They were frustrated because they weren't seeing that "one thing" they had set in their minds as the end-all, be-all of their journey. This is where I ask them, "If you never see change in that 'one thing' but have all these other incredible benefits, are the changes you're making still worth it?" And every time, they answer, "Yes, it is still worth it." Our frustrations are usually indicative of misplaced priorities and not an indicator of failure. The more you work on your health because you enjoy being healthy, the more you will forget your frustrations and embrace the process. There is no finish line, so take time to have fun along the way.

The old me keeps resurfacing, and it's hard to resist old patterns. There are aspects of our identities that we think are concrete, but we are not the finished product yet. We aren't a completed sculpture but rather a bit of clay still being shaped. As long as we keep working on ourselves, we are still malleable. I love this excerpt from C.S. Lewis: "Every time you make a choice, you are turning the central part of you, the part of you that chooses, into something a little different than it was before. And taking your life as a whole, with all your innumerable choices, all your life long, you are slowly turning this central thing into a heavenly creature or a hellish creature." Choose the new you daily. The choices will be in front of you to either revert back or press on. The danger isn't in choosing the old you. The greatest risk is feeling powerless to choose the new you. Ask yourself which path will get you closer to the creature you want to be. You don't have to beat the old you before you can be the new you. Victory comes when you choose the new you, even when the old you is the loudest.

THE HACK IN ACTION

One of my clients, Martin, was recently in Colorado for a work trip. The group he was with wanted to go for a hike up a nearby mountain. It ended up being a seven-mile round-trip hike. Out of the six who started out, only two made it to the top of the mountain. Martin was one of those two. Rewind one year, and he would not have been able to make that hike.

When Martin first reached out to me, he said he wanted to try making some changes, but I could tell he didn't believe in himself. Months later, he confirmed that by telling me that he had been afraid of starting again just to fail again. He had a pattern of starting from a place of guilt and shame, only to give up from that same place of guilt and shame. Martin had lost weight through restrictive dieting before but had always gained it back when life got stressful. He works in a demanding profession and often travels. He used junk food as a coping mechanism and alcohol most nights to unwind and get to sleep. These habits were not sustainable.

When we first started working together, he was self-conscious of his weight and did not want to step on a scale. We started small and practical. We forgot about weight and made lifestyle choices his main focus. A month into helping him with his nutrition, Martin wanted me to be his strength training coach, too. He gave up the high-intensity group fitness classes that he was doing from a place of self-punishment. He embraced (reluctantly, for sure) a different approach to self-care, not eating based on feelings, seeing exercise as a positive experience, and not using alcohol as a method of stress relief. The months that followed paid off big time. Seven months in, Martin was training hard regularly, tracking food when we needed to in his program, averaging twelve thousand steps per day, and starting to jog.

You are a living, breathing testament to what you have endured and what you can achieve.

I will never forget the day he messaged me to say he had jogged for an entire mile for the first time in his life. That was all him … he set that target for himself, and the excitement was so evident when he conquered that goal. A month later, he hiked to the top of a mountain and didn't stop when others gave up and turned back. Martin went from someone who saw running as drudgery and exercise as punishment to someone who found joy in tackling new challenges. He went from living in shame and using food and alcohol to cope with stress to knowing how to fuel his body and liking how he looked in photos.

What you start with will probably be what you finish with. If you start from a place of insufficiency and rely on self-defeating cycles, you will probably end up feeling insufficient and self-defeated. Do you want to be celebrating on the mountain and proud of achieving your goals or do you want to be at the bottom, saying, "What if?" or "Maybe one of these days?" The only way to achieve lasting victory is to love what your body can do but never settle for how you used to do it.

\|—\|

Cherish the small wins and milestones along the way. Celebrate the days when you push a little harder, run a bit farther, or lift a pound more. These are the building blocks of lasting change. You are more than your reflection in the mirror. You are a living, breathing testament to what you have endured and what you can achieve. Love your body for its strength, its ability to heal, and its unyielding ability to bounce back. Embrace the journey and know that every step forward, no matter how small, is a beautiful celebration of who you are becoming.

When things get hard, remember this: You are seeing a roadblock you never would have seen before. You were at the bottom of the mountain, the path was paved, and there were guardrails. But you've progressed, you've built the aptitude to climb higher than you ever could have before. Now you're hitting the rocky path. There are new obstacles you couldn't see from where you used to be. The struggle is a sign of the success of what you're doing. The more you can handle, the more challenging the terrain. But that just means you have entirely new challenges to explore. What once felt hard now feels easy. Look back and see how far you've truly come.

FOCUS ON BETTER, NOT PERFECT

Ditch the All-or-Nothing ... Once and for All

There's no problem so awful that you can't add some guilt to it and make it even worse.
— BILL WATTERSON, AUTHOR OF THE
CALVIN AND HOBBES COMICS

THE PROBLEM: WE HAVE AN ALL-OR-NOTHING MINDSET ABOUT HEALTH

TELL ME IF you've been here before: You're a few days into a new health initiative when you realize you slipped a bit, missed some targets, or forgot to complete a task. Your brain quickly shifts from guilt to resignation: "You already screwed up, so why even try now?" You spiral. You fall back into old comfort patterns and tell yourself you'll get back to it tomorrow. And the next day comes, and the last thing you want to do is face your choices from yesterday or feel like a failure again. Within a few days, your health initiative falls completely out of the back of your mind.

Or maybe you've been here: You decide enough is enough, and now is the time. You buy all the equipment. You cut out all the [insert demonized food group of choice here]. You make a plan to hit a workout seven days a week. You jump straight into the deep end because sink-or-swim is all you know. But a few weeks in, the burnout hits. Or an injury hits. Or life hits. Your plan is unsustainable, and you decide this lifestyle just "doesn't work for me." Well, not until about eight months later, and then you repeat the entire cycle again.

Both of these scenarios are examples of the "all-or-nothing" approach to fitness. This approach kills more hopeful ambitions than any other issue. There is no greater danger than expecting perfection in an area of inexperience. Perfectionism kills progress. We think we must be perfect to start, perfect to see progress, and perfect to sustain our new choices. The pressure of perfection delays the start. It creates false expectations of what progress will look like, and it detracts from the fun of the process.

Would you quit your job if you had one slightly off day? Of course not! You know you can bounce back the next day and that your job is essential to your lifelong goals. What if you approached your job like you do your health goals? You would not expect to keep a job for long or to be paid for work you never completed because you were waiting for everything to line up perfectly. Perfectionism can be paralyzing and demotivating. When we focus solely on achieving per-fection, we can become overwhelmed by the pressure to do everything perfectly and may be unable to start or complete tasks. This can lead to procrastination, missed opportuni-ties, and a sense of frustration and disappointment.

A more subtle sign of perfectionism in your health journey is when you become too eager to bypass the novice stage. It is so easy to see advanced strategies from people much further along than you and assume that you should be following what they are doing. This is what I like to call "skill skipping." There are layers of skills that will help you along your journey. It might feel like your progress speeds up when you skip to advanced strategies and techniques, but I assure you, you will miss essential skill development that will hinder you down the line.

A good example within weight-lifting is exercise form. Many beginners want to progress too quickly with weights and neglect developing a strong foundation. In the long run, this is far more dangerous and limiting than going more slowly at the start. It is much easier for me to teach someone the correct form on a barbell squat than to correct poor form that has been ingrained for many sessions. Skill skipping will cost you far more over a longer time horizon. It is easy to assume advanced strategies are better, but they aren't. Advanced means advanced, not better. The best strategy for a beginner is to start at the beginning. You can't skip the beginner stages and expect to find sustainability.

There is no lasting victory in all-or-nothing approaches to your health. Pursuing results at all costs will leave more scars than wins. Aiming for perfection will cause you to feel like a failure. Prioritizing speed by skill skipping will create gaps that are much harder to fill later. It's time to ditch the all-or-nothing … once and for all.

THE HACK: FOCUS ON BETTER, NOT PERFECT

Results often come in chunks. You can be doing everything correctly and notice no changes at all for several weeks. This is the point where many people pull back or change course. But when you stick it out, the results will often start showing in rapid succession. The all-or-nothing model never lasts long enough to produce winning in chunks. The better, not perfect, approach is the ideal strategy to compound your efforts into a system of wins.

Think of your fitness journey as your place of residence. You could have a home that feels warm and inviting. Or you could have one that is perfect in every way but makes people walk on eggshells. Which sounds more enjoyable? You would rather live in a vibrant, joy-filled home than a perfectly put-together house. The same is true for your health routines. There is no need for a "perfect" health plan that places inconvenience on everyone in your life or impossible standards on yourself.

Almost monthly, I give extra encouragement to some clients after they feel like they "messed up." One example is from a client named Emily, who would beat herself up mentally when her weight increased a little or when she was slightly off on her macronutrient targets. We worked out a calorie range instead of a specific number. That helped, but it was still not enough. We implemented an 80/20 rule that she felt good about. Basically, 80 percent of the days she needed to be perfectly in that range. Any days off up to 20 percent of the days (six days per month), she had to give herself grace and move on. Anything above 20 percent, we talked over and worked through on our weekly check-ins.

We also started having her check her weight more regularly—three times per week—but she only recorded the weekly average. The goal was to lower the pressure on each weigh-in and see the patterns over the long run without fixating on the week-to-week numbers. This helped her see that weight fluctuations were normal and that her weekly averages were moving in the direction we wanted. She learned. She grew. And still saw results and had more joy. This was from following a better, not perfect, strategy for her nutrition and for result tracking. The all-or-nothing model focuses on the result, but the better, not perfect, model puts the focus on the process. For far too long, results have been the centerpiece of conversations around health.

The most egregious culprit has been weight loss. The past seventy years of health narratives have led us to a place where weight looms so large in how so many people feel about themselves. I hope we can stop focusing on weight. In Hack 6, we talked about setting exercise goals that have nothing to do with the scale. Let's expand on that concept. We need to deemphasize weight as the primary metric of health and instead include it as one of many data points, along with height, age, cognitive function, lean body mass, body fat percentage, strength, sleep quality, gut health, mobility, flexibility, and endurance. When we do this, we unload all the pressure that sits on that number. This is where the better, not perfect, model thrives.

Progress isn't always linear. Growth isn't always measurable, at least not in the moment. Let me get nerdy for a second. One of my favorite thinkers is a German philosopher named G.W.F. Hegel (maybe you know the Hegelian Dialectic). His ideas pushed the philosophy of idealism. His theory of the human story can be summed up as an inevitable progression of human society to a more ideal situation. We still feel the impact of this idea today.

Society still holds an expectation that things, once on an upward trajectory, will continue that upward movement. If a stock price is rising, of course it will continue to rise. If you get a promotion at work, you assume that you will get another promotion down the road. But if we reflect on the situation, we know from experience that many fluctuations, periods of regression, and unforeseen challenges are on the path to any goal. Our brains are wired to see these as setbacks and unfortunate instances. Instead, we can reconfigure our mindset to accept that progress doesn't always keep going and to anticipate the ups and downs.

How do we begin this process? One measurement alone won't work. You need a set of criteria to determine "progress." Within this set, you need mental, emotional, physical, and personal criteria to assess how you are moving closer to meeting your goals. Stop using a single measurement like weight, inches, income, score, or grade to determine your growth or worth. Don't use one metric to determine progress. Instead, find as many metrics as possible. Compare and track the trajectory of each metric over time, and you will start to see wins piling up and leading to big health.

The goal of better, not perfect, is to keep you moving and progressing, even when you feel like you have stalled. The purpose is to be concrete instead of abstract, to build off of skills, not feelings. Aim for discipline, not perfect. Discipline is empowering, and it builds resilience and self-efficacy. Discipline encourages us to take action, even when we don't feel like it, and to make progress through consistent effort and determination. Do what you can today to make tomorrow easier.

WHAT YOU CAN DO TOMORROW

- **Make simple swaps.** Complexity challenges our balance. Simplicity changes our behavior. When trying to live better, not perfect, start with simplicity. You can add complexity over time as you acquire new skills. When it comes to swapping, start simple and swap a junk food snack for a high-protein snack. Swap a run that you dread for a nice walk. Swap watching TV on the couch for a stretch session on the floor. Swap one highly processed meal for one made with whole foods. Swap one high-calorie drink for plain tea, coffee, or water. Swap time scrolling on your phone for deep breathing, meditation, or prayer. If you can consciously make these simple swaps across your day, each choice will get easier over time and carry over into larger patterns of behavior.

- **Audit what feels hard.** Audit the tasks you resist doing. If you resist doing them despite knowing they are beneficial, there is unnecessary difficulty somewhere in the process. Here is the goal: remove at least some friction that makes the task harder than it needs to be. This strategy comes from Dan Charnas and his book *Work Clean*. How does it work?

  Step 1: List three tasks you find difficult. Choose one physical task, one digital task, and one complex process or errand. For our scenario, let's have the physical task be meal prepping, the digital task be meal tracking, and the complex process be meal planning for the week.

  Step 2: For each task, list one action you can take to decrease resistance or friction. Here are suggestions from Charnas: for physical tasks, arrange your space more effectively to make the task easier. For digital tasks, look for ways to automate part of the task or use software to simplify it. For complex processes, make a checklist of every step and keep it handy to use every time you begin the process. So, for our physical task of meal prepping, we would have an organized system of containers designated for our on-the-go meals. For meal tracking, we would spend one hour (just once) saving our favorite food items that we eat over and over to the app for quick tracking in the future. And for meal planning, we would create a checklist of items we know we use every week, as well as a list of favorite easy-prep meals. You will put in time on the front end but save that time and friction for weeks and months to come. You'll be amazed at how taking these proactive steps will simplify the tasks you find too difficult right now.

- **Create levels for your goals.** Your health goals are ambitious, but they are often too big to tackle all at once. Create attainable levels that build up to your goals and give you a growing sense of mastery. Imagine you were trying to learn a dance, trying to make a shelf in woodworking, or working on any other task that takes practice and skill. Break down the goal into smaller pieces and take them piece by piece. Don't try to take on too much too quickly. In the beginning stages of your fitness changes, less is more. Let's say you want to exercise five times per week. That's a great goal, but how likely is it that you'll go from zero workouts per week to five and sustain that in the long term? Highly unlikely. How could you create levels for this goal? Maybe in the first month, you work out three times a week. In the second month, you aim for four workouts per week but are still happy if you only get three. Once it feels easy to do four workouts per week, repeat what you did in the second month. There is no reason to rush and take on too much right away. Embrace the beginner stage. You are only a beginner once. When you are a beginner, you get more benefits from less work than in the later stages of your journey.

- **Talk yourself into it.** We are good at talking ourselves into things that aren't good for us. And we are really good at talking ourselves out of doing good things for ourselves. We come up with excuses, invent obstacles, and put our needs on the back burner. We need to counteract those actions with affirming language that empowers us to do what we know we need to do. Practice the skill of talking yourself into things you need to do but don't want to. Instead of talking yourself into one more show before bed, talk yourself into going to sleep on time. Instead of talking yourself into ordering takeout, talk yourself into eating the healthy meal that you prepared in advance. Many of the results you are looking for are hiding in these subtle mental shifts.

Here is the process: 1) Restate why this is a better option for you. 2) Reframe the task as a privilege you get to experience, not a chore you must endure. 3) Review how you feel later when

> Discipline encourages us to take action, even when we don't feel like it, and to make progress through consistent effort and determination.

you follow through. The better you get at talking yourself into decisions that are good for you, the easier it will be to see how much better you become at following through.

BUILDING MOMENTUM

The better, not perfect, model is a momentum-building mechanism. Doing what you can do, to the best of your ability and when you can do it, will lead to a higher capacity of achievement and resilience. Over time, your default state, the place where things feel simple and easy, will be at a higher level than your former baseline. Better, not perfect, is about gradually elevating your baseline so that what once felt hard will feel simple. This is true momentum. This is true sustainability. This is how you will see wins that you were never even anticipating before setting off on this journey.

STEP 1: Activate the Periphery Principle.

The Periphery Principle is what I call the process of unlocking unforeseen benefits simply by maintaining actions that have no downsides. Economists talk about the idea of positive and negative externalities. These are unintended costs or benefits from an economic activity that impact an uninvolved third party. For example, the renovation of a historical landmark near your home could increase the property value of your house. Within health and fitness, I see this periphery benefit play out in many ways. A great example is when you switch to a standing desk. You might swap to a standing desk to increase your daily calorie burn, which will happen. A periphery benefit could be that your hamstrings stay looser and you have less lower back pain. You might switch to a higher-protein diet because you're trying to build more muscle, which is a great approach. A likely periphery benefit is that you will have reduced hunger between meals and snack less during the day. Maybe you join a gym to have a place to exercise, but you end up meeting several like-minded individuals who become friends and part of your new healthy network.

The great thing about the Periphery Principle is that you can find wins without feeling like you have to exert energy toward them. Stockpile as many actions as you can that do not have any downside, and then see what kind of wins roll in by default. You can see potential opportunities open up to you that you might never have seen otherwise. This book exists due to the Periphery Principle. I was a guest on a podcast to talk about health and wellness, and my episode was heard by the right person at the right time. The same type of unintended benefits can come your way, but only if you do the work first.

STEP 2: Focus on sustainability.

What healthy options already feel easy for you? Do more of those activities. Eat more of those foods. You can build your sustainable plan around the sustainable habits you already have, not in spite of them. Don't spend a second trying to force yourself into what someone says is "optimal." People will ask me what the ideal training split is for muscle gain, and my answer is always, "Whichever training plan you can stick to and see progress over time." Don't waste any energy toward approaches that require 100 percent adherence or perfection. That's not sustainable. Sickness happens. Family events happen. Circumstances beyond your control happen. Sustainability is as much about flexibility as it is about consistency. Once your plan is sustainable, you won't be afraid of a trip or vacation, rest days, weekends, social gatherings, new hurdles, life events, plateaus, or next steps.

STEP 3: Abandon guilt.

I know I talked about guilt in the last Hack, but it is worthwhile to discuss guilt again in terms of the better, not perfect, approach. Think back to the Periphery Principle. Guilt also works as an example, but only as a negative one. The unintended negative consequences of guilt can be almost limitless. It is impossible to predict the depths that guilt can pull you if not kept in check. There is not even a single positive side effect of guilt that gives it a redeeming quality. If you make a mistake, own it and fix it. If you hurt someone else, apologize and correct your behavior. If you harm yourself, forgive yourself and love what your body can do. No aspect of your fitness and health journey will improve with guilt sprinkled in. Thinking of the Calvin and Hobbes quote at the start of this chapter, I would add: "There is no win so great that you can't add some guilt to it and make it obsolete." If you slip up, which you definitely will, in your health plan, the important thing is to get right back on track. Guilt spirals only push you further away from a healthy mindset and healthy actions.

STEP 4: Pursue adventure.

Adventure is for everyone. I believe we were designed with a thirst for adventure. And the best part is that adventure comes in many shapes and sizes. No template exists for adventure. What excites you? What hobbies, interests, passions, or creative work do you want to pursue? How can that interest play alongside your health and either help you attain your health goals or drive you to take better care of yourself? No one can create adventure for you; you have to create it for yourself. Pair your hobbies with your health to experience a renewed passion for taking care of yourself that goes beyond looks or meeting someone else's expectations. Are you actively finding ways to challenge yourself, pursuing actions that foster a sense of joy, exploring new possibilities, reading big ideas, and dreaming up "impossible" goals? Get creative. Foster a sense of adventure and play. And have fun!

REMOVING OBSTACLES

Here are a few common concerns for this Hack and how to address them.

Where do I start when it all feels hard? The worst place to be is overwhelmed and second-guessing. This is when you must tap into your reserve. Think back: What did you once have working for you that you dropped the ball on? That's a great place to start because you have a bedrock of proof in that area. Think now. Who do you have in your contact sphere who is a little further along or a little more disciplined than you? This is the best person to ask for guidance or suggestions. Think forward. What can you cut out of your life for a time that will make things feel easier? Sometimes, we are too focused on what we need to add and forget that the easiest change can be to get rid of something that isn't working for us.

How do I keep from falling back into the all-or-nothing approach? You probably have years of hardwiring trying to pull you back into the all-or-nothing model. It's likely your default state, but now you are trying to rewire your default. This is not a passive process. You cannot "accidentally" switch from all-or-nothing to the better, not perfect, mindset. It is a daily choice. You choose to flip that mental switch more days than not until it becomes your new default state. Use the better, not perfect, approach here too. Can you choose to flip that switch more often? Can you be better at activating an externally driven and internally forgiven mindset for your health and well-being strategies?

How do I set more health targets when what I really care about is my weight? I do not want to demonize weight loss or weight gain. There are many instances when weight gain or loss is needed. But fixating only on weight is almost always counterproductive. You cannot make your weight go down or up. You can only control certain levers of behavior that are likely to impact weight gain or loss. You will be far better off controlling the controllables and tracking and measuring the levers that you can adjust daily than putting all your focus on an internal biologic mechanism that you cannot directly manipulate. Setting activity targets, sleep targets, hydration targets, nutrition targets, mindfulness targets, and effort targets will benefit far more than just a weight target because they give you actionable steps to take along the way to larger objectives.

What do I do when I'm doing the right things but not seeing any changes? Have you ever given money to charity? If so, did you track your every dollar and demand to see an exact accounting of every specific result that your money produced? No, you didn't. You gave to an organization you trusted with a mission you support. You gave to give, not to receive. Imagine investing in your health as a charitable donation. You give energy, time, and attention to yourself (the organization you trust) to support your well-being (the mission you support). You will never have a one-to-one printout of inputs to outputs. Almost all of the important work is happening behind the scenes. Do what you already know is good for your body and try to do it better and better over time. If you are not sure what is good for you or how to onboard more good options, hire a trusted health professional to create a plan for you until you know you can sustain it on your own. Remember that doing good things for yourself with no visible results is always better than doing no good things for yourself that have either no visible results or visibly poor results.

Nothing (and no one) is stopping you unless you let it.

THE HACK IN ACTION

Bekah was your classic overachiever. She was a special education teacher and social media creator, and she was starting her own business as a young mom. It is safe to say that her stress levels were high, even on a good day. With everything she had going on, Bekah still thought she should be able to do it all, all the time.

Bekah started training with me, and it was clear that her biggest battle wasn't not doing enough. It was trying to do too much. Her adrenal system was worn out, and her mental health was not ideal—and her body showed it through

197

illness, poor sleep, and little response to training or fat loss. Results were slow to show up for our first six months. Bekah was great at juggling it all, at least for three to four days or even one to two weeks. But then the buildup of fatigue and stress would inevitably sidetrack her consistency.

Over and over, we came back to her all-or-nothing mindset. Bekah started to push back against the mom guilt, the health guilt, and the negative self-talk, and she made simple swaps she could stick to, even on the toughest days. Guess what? The results that had been so hard to find started rolling in. Better sleep, better stress management, better consistency with balanced meals, less alcohol, and more self-care snowballed into visible mental and physical results.

The change was dramatic. I recently asked Bekah to share what changes she made that helped her become the new version of herself. Bekah's ideas might help other people like her. Her thoughts were very enlightening, so I am sharing them in full here:

> *"I realized I owe it to myself to spend just as much time, effort, and energy on myself as I spend on everyone else. I realized I don't have to settle for 'good enough.' I realized I'm the only person whose validation actually matters to me. I realized I don't have to wait on someone else to make the positive changes that I knew needed to be made. It was mostly a mindset shift: I deserve more."*

Bekah is a different person from when I first met her. She is the first person to share how shocked she is to see the new version of herself. It didn't come from special supplements, a secret workout plan, or a fat-loss fad. It came because she got the mental game under control and let her actions follow. She put more energy into taking care of herself than trying to please other people and live life based on their expectations. Bekah's story is reflective of an essential truth: nothing (and no one) is stopping you unless you let it. You won't believe who you can become until you're already well on the path, so start now.

⊪—⊪

The better, not perfect, model is about knowing who you are and then finding small ways to improve yourself. What if you committed to slow improvement over the next one to three years? You'd be unstoppable with a clear plan of action and a long-term mindset. I say this with every bit of compassion and sincerity that I can: You get to choose, and it's not too late to turn things around. It's time to act. Vaclav Havel, a Czech anti-Soviet dissident and politician, said, "Vision is not enough, it must be combined with venture. It is not enough to stare up the steps, we must step up the stairs." Be bold in how you begin. Start climbing. Strive to be better, not perfect, and you will see your health dramatically improve bit by bit.

THE FINAL WORD

Whatever you can do, or dream you can,
begin it. Boldness has genius, power,
and magic in it. Begin it now.
— W.H. MURRAY, MOUNTAINEER AND WRITER

RECENTLY WENT BACK and read my master's thesis. Two years of coursework plus an entire semester of focused research went into producing my culminating project on the impact students had on school culture in late imperial Russia. I showed that while the Russian authorities wanted the state schools to support the official aims of the state, the students and their families had agency to turn the benefits of education toward their own ends. This is probably not the most fascinating topic to you, but I felt I was contributing a new perspective to the history of education.

Hundreds of hours of research and writing paid off when I passed my verbal defense and won awards for my efforts. But that paper has probably been read by less than thirty people ever. This book has been a similar labor of love, but

I certainly hope it has a wider audience than thirty people. I know the topics of health and fitness appeal to only part of the population, but my primary purpose is to communicate my passion and hopefulness that you can live a healthy, happy, and balanced life.

The quality of our lives is curated by what we say yes to and what we say no to. If you only take one thing away from this book, I want it to be this: You always have the opportunity to say yes to the healthier version of you. You make choices every day that shape your physical, mental, and spiritual health. You make mistakes. You are human, after all. But you can always be better today than you were yesterday, and that will come by making better choices. Find the small wins and build habits that align with who you aspire to be. The prouder you are of your choices, the easier the path to sustainable health becomes.

Be encouraged! My prayer and hope for you is that you find encouragement in your health journey and are surrounded by a supportive community. If you benefited from this book in big or small ways, I would be thrilled to hear about your wins.

Keep winning small,
Bryan Holyfield

ABOUT THE AUTHOR

BRYAN HOLYFIELD is married to his high school sweetheart, Hannah. They met as missionary kids whose families were serving in Moscow, Russia. Together, they are raising their four sons to be men of character and faith. Bryan has a bachelor's degree in Secondary Social Sciences and a master's in Russian and East European Studies. He was a successful social studies teacher and soccer coach before he founded Holyfit Coaching and transitioned into full-time fitness and nutrition coaching. Bryan is a Certified Personal Trainer through NFPT and a Certified Nutrition Coach through Precision Nutrition. Bryan played soccer in college but let fatherhood, education, and career get in the way of protecting his health. He suffered a low-back injury in his late twenties that made him realize he needed to start taking better care of his body to be able to be the man and father he wanted to be. When the COVID-19 pandemic hit three years later, he saw so many colleagues and friends allow their health to suffer. Bryan knew he had the experience and communication skills to have an impact on a great number of people.

He is passionate about building strong and healthy leaders to the glory of God with a global and missional impact. Outside of work, Bryan stays active by coaching his sons' sports teams, hiking, duck hunting, playing soccer and disc golf, and serving as a leader in his local church. If you ever need to know about the best coffee or hiking in North Georgia, Bryan has the inside scoop for you.

Connect with Bryan Holyfield

Website: holyfitcoaching.com/smallwins
Instagram: instagram.com/bryanholy.fit/
Podcast on Spotify: *Winning Small* with Bryan Holyfield
LinkedIn: www.linkedin.com/in/holyfit

ACKNOWLEDGMENTS

FIND IT DIFFICULT to credit everyone who has challenged and supported me during the process of writing and publication. This has been a labor of love, and it would have been impossible without the constant encouragement, feedback, and check-ins from an amazing community. I would like to express my heartfelt thanks to:

My Family

My wife deserves all the credit for taking on extra roles within our family during the late nights and weekends spent writing this book. Hannah, I cannot express how much your love, patience, and encouragement have meant to me during this season! Our sons are too young to really understand what it means to write a book, but they tried their best to keep noise levels down when it was writing time. Notice I said "tried." I love you guys with everything in me.

To my parents, siblings, in-laws, and extended family, thank you for your belief and excitement for this project. You all mean the world to me.

My Friends

Thank you for your constant encouragement, motivation, and willingness to listen to my ideas and provide valuable feedback. Your belief in me kept me going. Mark, Stephen, and Jerry, meeting with you guys every week for prayer and accountability is incredibly life-giving. Thank you for your friendship!

Readers and Testers

To those who volunteered as testers and provided valuable feedback, thank you for your time and dedication. Your input helped shape this book into what it is today.

Publishing Team

A special thank you to the entire team at Times 10 Publications. Your professionalism and support made this process a delight.

My Clients

I'm grateful to my clients who have been on this journey with me every step of the way. I love the community and friendships we've built. And I want to thank many of them who allowed their stories to be shared in this book. Your efforts to change your health and to encourage me in the writing process have been a constant source of inspiration.

The Readers

Last but not least, to you, the reader. Thank you for investing your time and resources into this book. I hope the Hacks I detailed here will give you a launching pad and momentum-builder in your health journey! This book would not have been possible without the support and contributions of each of you. Thank you for being a part of this incredible journey.

With gratitude,
Bryan Holyfield

SNEAK PEEK

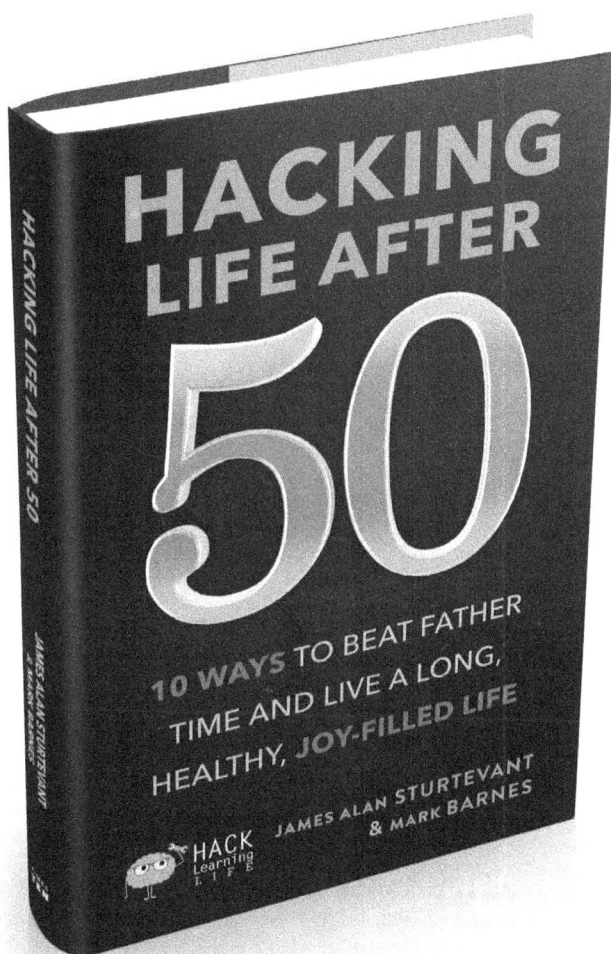

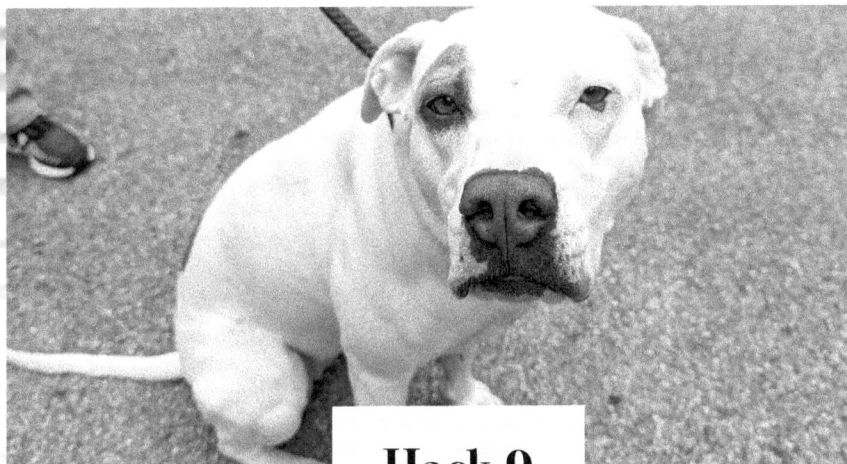

Hack 9

CONNECT

You're not done making friends

*The most terrible poverty is loneliness
and the feeling of being unloved.*
— MOTHER TERESA, FOUNDER OF
MISSIONARIES OF CHARITY

THE PROBLEM: YOU'RE FEELING ISOLATED

LIFE AFTER FIFTY can be lonely. This is not only sad, but it can also be dangerous. The Centers for Disease Control and Prevention, in an online article titled "Loneliness and Social Isolation Linked to Serious Health Conditions," equated social isolation's health impact to standard villains of longevity such as smoking and obesity. This is a sobering claim. It's time to recognize that isolation, aside from being tragic, is also a threat to health.

Think of all the events that can happen after age fifty that accelerate this isolation:

- Your kids leave home.

- You retire and then miss your coworkers.

- You lose physical mobility, so you aren't as active.

- A relationship dissolves.

- A dear friend moves to be close to their kids.

- Your aged parent dies.

- A beloved sibling dies.

- Your friends start to die.

- Your dog dies.

- Your spouse dies.

- Your familiar neighborhood doesn't seem familiar anymore because your friends are downsizing and moving away.

This list was so easy to make and not meant to be exhaustive. It could go on and on. One of the cruelest aspects to aging is that, as you get older, these isolating factors grow exponentially. When you reminisce about aging and deceased friends and family, you start to wonder, *Will I be the last one standing?* In this life stage, attending and planning memorial services become a painful reality.

One factor that can exacerbate feelings of isolation and loneliness, not to mention envy, is social media. We know many contemporaries who doom-scroll on Facebook almost nightly. They peruse self-promotional posts from acquaintances who seem to have it all. They're off on magnificent vacations, their beautiful families arrange themselves perfectly for group photos at celebrations and holidays, and their carefully selected photos and profile pics make them look twenty years younger.

Please understand that there's probably lots of drama hidden behind these highly scripted and curated billboards of domestic bliss. They likely aren't nearly as content, and their families nearly as congenial, as they look. Your nightly Facebook journeys could, unfortunately, act as painful reminders of everything you don't have and everything you aren't. Such emotions can contribute to feelings of isolation. But we don't want to come off as hypocrites in terms of social media. We've posted self-promotionally. It's fun to share photos you're proud of and have friends celebrate your achievement. Social media also has wonderful aspects and can reunite lost friends and foster new relationships, but we've come to recognize the negative side of these powerful tools. These platforms should serve us, not make us feel bad. We can help you use social media in ways that serve you.

"Social media does have the power to facilitate new relationships and nurture old ones. A great tactic is to utilize direct messaging. My favorite DM strategies are to send a congratulation when a friend shares an accomplishment (even if I'm a little envious) and a condolence when a friend faces a hardship or loss. My experience has been that such messages make the recipients feel good and lead to more interactions between them and me. That's a great use of social media."

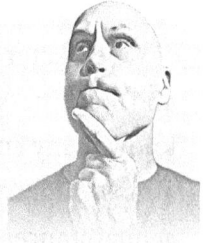

Coming to grips with the bitter realities of this life stage and dealing with feelings of envy that everyone else is thriving because of what they post on social media is hard enough. What's doubly challenging is to figure out how to break out of your After-50s isolation and rejoin the world. If you're retired, you've lost the social interaction opportunity that came by default at work each day. If you're not retired, you know what to expect in your not-too-distant future. Are you cognizant that the extensive social network you interact with daily will dwindle to a trickle? What preparations are you making for this loss? The previous sentence articulates what we'll attempt to do in this Hack.

Meeting and socializing with people probably happened organically for most of your life. You met people at work. You met people at church. You met people through your kid's activities. You became friends with your neighbors who were at a similar life stage. Now that you're after fifty, it's important for you to be intentional about connecting. The same skill sets you utilized when you were younger to find the right job or the right spouse can now be resurrected and then adapted to the goal of finding new friends. The great news is that, compared to interviewing for a job or proposing to a potential spouse, finding new friends after fifty is a low-stakes aspiration. If you attempt to connect with a new friend and the interaction fizzles, you're out virtually nothing and you can learn a lot about how to improve your search filter. And, you're not attempting to find just one dream job or just one soulmate. There's a lot less pressure when you're just trying to interact with more people and find new friends.

THE HACK: CONNECT

It's helpful to think about connection as capital. When economists talk about capital, they're referring to assets. Acquiring new friends *is* acquiring new assets. New friends are valuable. They can make you happier and healthier. They can be there for you in a crisis. You can be as beneficial to them as they are to you. We have plenty of friends who are contemporaries and consider us as assets. So we're going to stick with our analogy.

As we mentioned in The Problem section of this Hack, our desire is to spark intentionality about connecting. That's not to say that new friendships cannot blossom organically; we just don't want you to sit idly by, waiting for someone else to make the first move. That probably didn't work decades ago at your high school dances unless, of course, you were smoking hot, and it probably won't work at this stage of life. We aim to give you some ideas, but we're more concerned with helping you find the motivation and the confidence to step out of your comfort zone and make the first move. We won't just yell, *Get over your fears and get out there!* Instead, we want to inspire you to get out there in your own time and in your own way.

To bond with others, you need to be approachable. Have you ever evaluated your approachability? Do you broadcast a welcoming vibe? Would you feel comfortable meeting you? These are important questions, and adjustments in this realm could be instrumental in achieving a broader social network.

As with all the Hacks in this book, we encourage you to create your own goals and your own roadmap to expand your connections—and we'll offer many suggestions along the way. This is ultimately your journey, but sometimes you need a nudge in the right direction. This Hack works hand-in-hand with Hack 8. Often, the pursuit of engagement leads to opportunities to expand your social interactions with like-minded people. As with engagement, networking is an invaluable tool.

And finally, even though the focus of this Hack is to grow your social network, you probably have more relationships than you think. Those bonds with friends and family need to be nurtured and maintained. Please don't take these important folks for granted.

WHAT YOU CAN DO TOMORROW

The loneliness that often accompanies life after fifty can be compared to a relationship breakup. The relationship in our analogy represents all the social interactions you had when you were younger. The breakup represents diminished opportunities to meet and greet as you sail past fifty. Most of us have experienced painful breakups. Trusted friends and family members nudged us back out into the dating pool. We needed those nudges. As awkward as it may seem to you, we're going to encourage you to put yourself back out there into the social interaction pool, too, and start forging new relationships.

- **Interact.** Typically, when you pursue engagement, you realize the potential for new social interaction. And, the folks you meet when engaged in an activity will probably be interested in the same things as you. You'll automatically have important commonalities. This is an essential ingredient for any budding friendship. Go back over your list of ideas of activities you'd like to try in pursuit of engagement. Then, consider how each could place you in a situation where you might meet new people. Consider how you'll respond if such a situation presents itself.

- **Chat with a stranger.** You may be reluctant to talk to people you don't know. The idea of it might make you uncomfortable. You might be worried that it's unsafe or you'll send the wrong message. If this suggestion is a bridge too far for you—we understand. But we are not talking about deep or intimate conversations. All we want you to do is get accustomed to smiling and saying *Hi* to people you don't know. You don't even have to break stride. If you make eye contact with someone at the grocery, just smile and greet them, and then you can keep on trucking. Or, if you walk into a building in front of someone, hold the door for them, whether they are male or female, and invite them out of the elements. If you're in line and ready to purchase an item, and you get a pleasant vibe from a line mate, ask them about an item they are purchasing. You may learn about a cool product. These interactions will help you reactivate social muscles that may have atrophied. These are short, low-stakes social excursions. What we love about doing this is that whether or not we get much back in return, chatting with strangers puts us in a better mood.

"I didn't used to be a very social person. I'd even avoid neighbors. After reading How to Talk to Anyone *by Leil Lowndes, I decided to take some chances and strike up conversations with people I'd bump into on walks. Lowndes's advice is to look for common points of interest and start there. I saw a neighbor gardening, and I stopped and joked that I had some gardening work she could do since hers was so beautiful and mine was hideous. This led to a lovely five-minute conversation and a neighbor I now speak to regularly."*

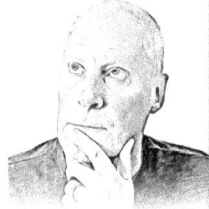

- **Interview a trusted friend.** Invite a dear friend to meet over coffee. Explain to them that you're going to pick their brain on a project that you're passionate about. After you've sat down, slurped some java, and caught up, tell them about your objective to have more social interaction, and ask if they can help you in this quest by answering some questions. Ask them about the origins of your relationship. Here are some suggestions:

- What was your first impression of me?
- What did we talk about early in our friendship?
- How did we meet?
- When did you first start to consider me a friend?
- How does my friendship serve you?
- How could I become a better friend to you?
- How could I become more approachable?
- Do you have any ideas on how I could meet people?
- Would you be willing to join me when I go on a new experience?

We love these questions. If you muster the courage to ask them, you may learn a lot about yourself in the process. Regardless, you and your friend will probably have a wonderful time reminiscing, and you'll strengthen the bond between you two.

- **Evaluate your employment status.** You need to start this process in earnest tomorrow. If you're working, start evaluating how long you want to work. Get serious about this question. The more specific you can get about when to retire, the more potential you'll have to exert some control over when and how it happens. Working or not working is a major factor regarding social interaction. Consider how you'll replace interactions with others when you retire. If you are retired, evaluate how you feel about not working when it comes to social interaction. If you have plenty of social interaction and are retired, congratulations! But many aren't so fortunate. Going back to work, working part time, or volunteering are options. If you're feeling isolated, spend time tomorrow considering these three options from the perspective of how they would impact social interaction.

- **Evaluate your living status.** While you're evaluating your working life, go ahead and evaluate your living situation as well. This one has the potential to be emotional, particularly if you've lived somewhere for a long time. Financial factors may trump any such evaluation, but tomorrow, just consider the following: *Is my living situation conducive*

SMALL WINS, BIG HEALTH

to social interaction? This is a challenging and important question. We both struggle on this front. We both live in large houses where we raised families. We have a deep sense of comfort and belonging in our homes. We invested equity and sweat equity in these houses. But do they still fit our purposes? Are our homes isolating us? Should we downsize? Should we move to a 55-plus community? Should we move to a new state? Questions about your working life or your living situation will probably not be answered right away, but you can start evaluating both in earnest tomorrow.

BUY
HACKING LIFE AFTER 50

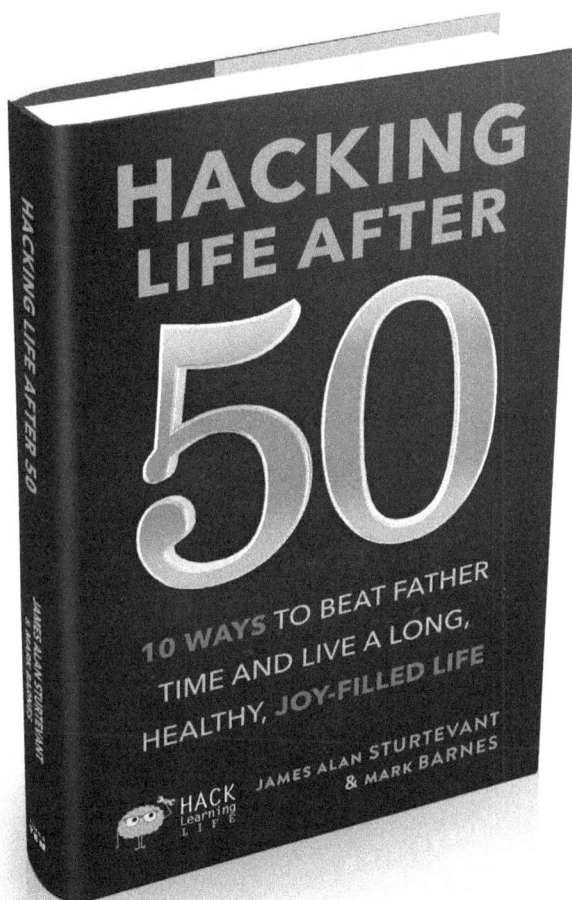

AVAILABLE AT:
Amazon.com
10Publications.com
and bookstores near you

MORE FROM
TIMES 10 PUBLICATIONS

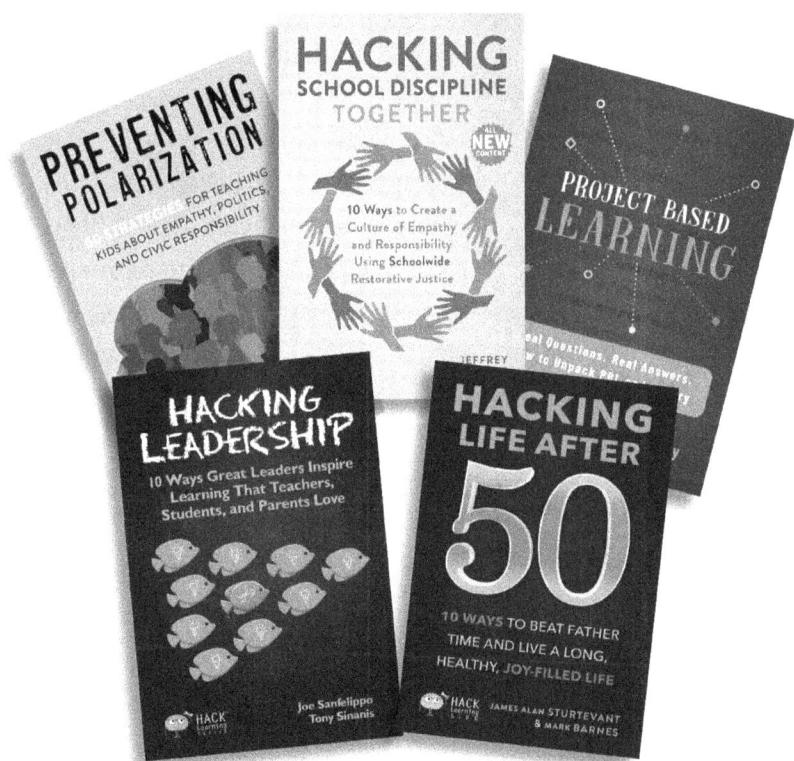

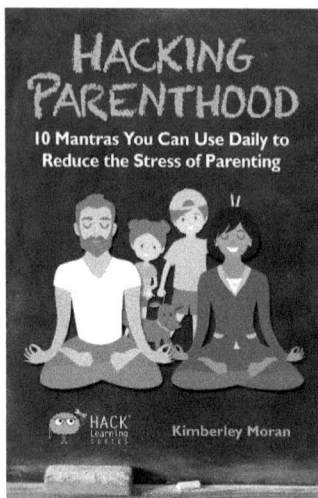

Hacking Parenthood
10 Mantras You Can Use Daily to Reduce the Stress of Parenting
Kimberley Moran

As a parent, you may throw out consequences willy-nilly and be frustrated with the daily chaos. Enter parent mantras, invaluable anchors wrapped in tidy packages that offer cues to stop and reset. These will become your go-to tools to calm your mind, focus your parenting, and concentrate on what you want for your kids. Simplify parenting and maximize communication while keeping your cool.

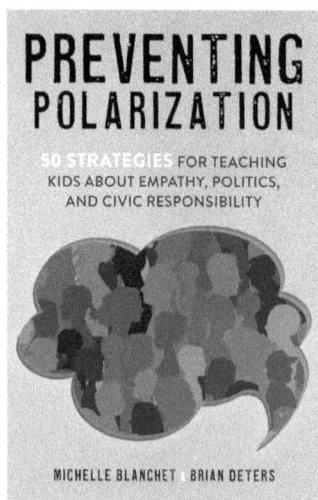

Preventing Polarization
50 Strategies for Teaching Kids About Empathy, Politics, and Civic Responsibility
Brian Deters and Michelle Blanchet

In an era that has become incredibly polarized, we can help our students learn how to come together despite differences and become active and engaged citizens. Ideally, education would equip students to care about the world and help them shape their futures. A one-off course on civics is not enough. These strategies create experiences to help students (and adults) break down barriers.

Lead With Grace
Leaning Into the Soft Skills of Leadership
Jessica Cabeen

Jessica Cabeen

Leaning into
the Soft Skills of Leadership

LEADFORWARD ▶▶

With technology, we interact with families, students, and staff 24/7, not just during the school day. Pressures can sway who we are into one who values online likes more than the authentic interactions that establish deep relationships. Teachers, principals, parents, and superintendents will be empowered to build confidence to lean into the soft skills of leadership and lead with grace.

Permission to Pause
A Journal for Teachers
Dorothy VanderJagt

PERMISSION
TO PAUSE

A Journal for Teachers

Dorothy VanderJagt

By giving yourself *Permission to Pause* for a few minutes each day, you gain clarity on your priorities and unravel what is worth nurturing and what you can let go. Journaling is an investment in yourself. This eighty-day journal with prompts will help you develop greater self-care and mindfulness, along with ideas for actions to become a more mindful educator.

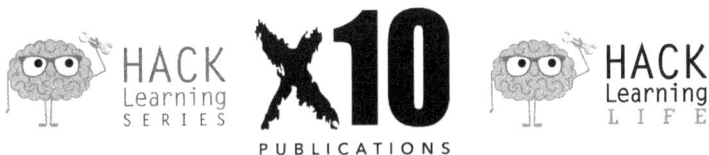

TIMES 10 PUBLICATIONS provides practical solutions that busy people can read today and use tomorrow. We bring you content from experienced researchers and practitioners, and we share it through books, podcasts, webinars, articles, events, and ongoing conversations on social media. Our books and materials help turn practice into action. Stay in touch with us at 10Publications.com and follow our updates @10Publications.

www.ingramcontent.com/pod-product-compliance
Lightning Source LLC
Chambersburg PA
CBHW062128020426
42335CB00013B/1146